MEDITERRANEAN DIET

Step by Step Guide and Proven Recipes for Smart Eating and Weight Loss

John Carter

The information herein is offered for informational purposes solely, and is universal as so. The presentation of the information is without contract or any type of guarantee assurance.

The trademarks that are used are without any consent, and the publication of the trademark is without permission or backing by the trademark owner. All trademarks and brands within this book are for clarifying purposes only and are the owned by the owners themselves, not affiliated with this document.

Table of Content

Introduction

I want to thank you and congratulate you for purchasing the book, *"Mediterranean Diet – Step By Step Guide And Proven Recipes For Smart Eating And Weight Loss"*.

This book contains proven steps and strategies on how to follow the Mediterranean diet properly, not just for the best results in weight loss but for optimum health too.

The Mediterranean diet is, without a doubt, the healthiest diet on earth. It is also one of the oldest and, as such, is proven to work. I will be explaining the principles of the Mediterranean diet to you in simple and easy to understand terms, along with tips on how to do the diet properly and how not to do it. I will also give you an easy reference list of the foods you can eat and those that you should avoid. Finally, I will finish off with some delicious recipes for you to try; I promise that, once you have tried them, you won't want to go back to your old way of eating! I will be showing you some wonderful breakfasts, a choice of soups and salads, main courses, a few delicious desserts and even some easy to prepare snacks.

Thanks again for purchasing this book, I hope you enjoy it!

Chapter 1: How Will the Mediterranean Diet Benefit You?

For many people, foods like lasagna, gyros, pizza, rack of lamb and loaves of white bread are what makes up the Mediterranean diet, most likely because this is what they eat when they visit a Mediterranean country. We tend to think of long, wine filled lunches, with many courses and this is what the original Mediterranean diet was like. However, the last 50 years or so have seen a huge change; Mediterranean meals have been pumped full of unhealthy fat and calories, pushing aside the traditional foods of the region. What used to be a very healthy and cheap way of eating is now firmly associated with a range of different diseases – obesity, heart disease, mood disorders, diabetes, and much more besides. And that's not to mention the fact that what used to be a healthy way of eating is now unhealthy and filled with heavy fatty dishes, at least for the tourist aspects. For the people who live in the Mediterranean, things are different.

When World War II had concluded, Ansel Keys from the Mayo Clinic studied the diets of around 13,000 men. All of them were middle-aged and they lived across the US, Italy, Japan, Greece, Finland, The Netherlands, and Yugoslavia. His conclusions were a revelation – American men, very well-fed, showed much higher heart disease rates than in any other country that had been struck by the rations and deprivations that took place during the war. The poorest people in Key's study were those men who lived on the Greek Island of Crete and they had, without any doubt, the best heart health of any of those studied. This was down to the physical work they did and their food pyramid, somewhat unique compared to the rest of the world.

The food pyramid for the Mediterranean diet is based on the diet traditions from the 1960's in Greece, Crete, and Southern Italy. This was a time when chronic disease was at its lowest level in these countries and life expectancy was much higher than anywhere in the world, despite having a very limited access to medical services. Their diet consisted of homegrown and fresh food but it wasn't just that – the Mediterranean people exercise daily, they share their meals with others and they fully appreciate the pleasure of eating the food they have.

8 Benefits of A Mediterranean Diet

The Mediterranean diet is loaded with benefits, not least the delicious foods and wine that you get to enjoy on a daily basis. These are the 8 main benefits of the diet:

1. Low Sugar and Low in Processed Foods

The Mediterranean diet consists mainly of natural foods and ingredients, such as legumes, olives oil, vegetables, fruits, unrefined cereals, and small amounts of animal products (preferably local sourced and organic). In contrast to a typical Western diet, it has little sugar in it and virtually free from GMO or other artificial ingredients, such as HFCS (high-fructose corn syrup). If you have a sweet tooth, the Mediterranean diet provides amply, with fruits, and homemade desserts that use honey for natural sweetness.

Aside from vegetation-based foods, the diet also has another staple – local caught fresh fish and small amounts of cheeses and yogurts made from sheep, cow, or goat milk. These provide an excellent and healthy way to get healthy fats and healthy cholesterol into your diet. Sardines, anchovies, and other similar fish are central to the diet and are eaten more than meat products. While the people of the Mediterranean are not vegetarian, the diet consists of small amounts only of meats and other heavier foods, opting instead for lighter and healthier meals that include fish. This is highly beneficial for those who want to shed some weight and improve their health in terms of heart health, cholesterol, and their intake of omega-3 fatty acids.

2. Lose Weight Healthily

The Mediterranean diet promotes healthy weight loss without leaving you hungry and helps you to maintain your new weight in a realistic and sustainable way for the rest of your life. The Mediterranean diet enjoys huge success around the whole world with people who want to lose weight as is helps you to reduce your intake of fat in a natural and easy way, thanks to the amount of nutrient-dense foods that you eat.

The Mediterranean diet is not a strict one and is open to a small measure of interpretation. Some people prefer to cut their carbs, their proteins or stay somewhere in the middle and that can be done on this diet as it focuses on consuming a good amount of healthy fat while keeping levels of carbohydrate intake low and increasing the intake of healthy proteins. If you prefer to eat more meat than legumes, that is fine because you will still lose weight without any sense of deprivation, eating a higher level of seafood and high quality dairy. All of these also provide other benefits in the form of probiotics and omeaga-3s.

Grass fed meats, dairy products, and wild caught fish contain good amounts of fatty acids that are essential to the working of the human body. They help you to feel fuller for longer, keep your blood sugar levels down and improve your energy and mood. If you prefer to eat more of a plant-based diet, you can get the same results with legumes and healthy whole grains, particularly those that have been soaked and sprouted.

3. Improves Your Heart Health

Research has shown that those who adhere to the Mediterranean diet, consuming plenty of omega-3 foods and monounsaturated fats, have a much lower mortality rate from heart disease. A diet that is rich in ALA (alpha-linolenic acid) found in olive oil, such as the Mediterranean diet, has been shown to have very high protective levels and can decrease the risk of death from cardiac arrest by up to 30% and the risk of sudden cardiac death by up to 45%.

Research carried out at the Warwick Medical School on blood pressure showed that when the levels were compared between those who ate a diet high in extra-virgin olive oil and those who consumed more sunflower oil, those on the olive oil had significantly lower blood pressure. This is because olive oil increases the bioavailability of nitric oxide and keeps your arteries clearer and more dilated.

4. Helps to Fight off Some Cancers

The European Journal of Cancer Prevention says that "the biological mechanisms for cancer prevention associated with the Mediterranean diet have been related to the favorable effect of a balanced ratio of omega-6 and omega-3 essential fatty acids and high amounts of fiber, antioxidants and polyphenols found in fruit, vegetables, olive oil and wine."
To quantify that, plant foods, in particular vegetables and fruits, are the basis of the Mediterranean diet and it is these foods that help to fight off cancer in virtually every single way. They do this because they are full of antioxidants, they protect your DNA from becoming damaged, they stop cells from mutating and they lower inflammation, as well as

slowing down the growth of tumors. There are a lot of studies that point to olive oil consumption as being a natural cure for cancer and for decreasing the risk of bowel and colon cancer. It could be that it has a protective effect on cancer cell development because of its propensity for reducing inflammation and reducing oxidative stress. It also helps to promote a healthy weight and better blood sugar balance.

5. Can Help to Treat or Prevent Diabetes

There is evidence to suggest that the Mediterranean diet helps to fight off inflammatory diseases, including type 2 diabetes and metabolic syndrome. The main reason why the Mediterranean diet is successful at preventing these diseases is because it controls insulin production. Insulin is a hormone that controls your blood sugar, and in many diets, is responsible for weight gain and a struggle to lose it, no matter how many diets we undertake.

By controlling blood sugar levels with the right balance of healthy whole foods, the body is able to burn off fat better and provide more energy. A diet that is low in sugar and high in fresh foods and healthy fats is a natural cure for diabetes. The American Heart Association says that the Mediterranean diet is actually higher in fat than a normal American diet but it is lower in levels of saturated fat. The diet is normally a ratio of about 40% complex carbohydrate, 30-40% healthy fat, and 20-30% high quality protein. This is the ideal balance for keeping your hunger and weight eves under control and for keeping the body in hormonal homeostasis, thus normalizing insulin levels.

The sugar in the diet comes mainly from wine, fruit, and the odd local dessert. Most people tend to drink water, coffee, and red wine, rather than the popular sodas and fizzy drinks consumed across the Western world as a whole. Some versions of the Mediterranean diet do contain carbohydrates in the form of pasta and bread but the activity levels and low sugar consumption of the diet also mean that resistance to insulin is rare, cutting out the dips and spikes in blood sugar that contribute towards diabetes.

Most people in the Mediterranean will eat a well-balanced breakfast within 2 hours of waking up. This helps to balance off their blood sugar when it as its lowest point. They will eat three filling meals a day, full of healthy fiber and fats and tend to have their largest meal at midday, rather than at night. Opposite to this is the standard American diet, which is composed of no breakfast, snacks throughout the day on high carbohydrate and high sugar foods and eating large meals at night when they are not active.

6. Help to Improve Mood and Cognitive Function

Studies show that the Mediterranean diet can help to treat diseases such as Parkinson's, Alzheimer's and dementia and can also slow the onset of these diseases. Cognitive disease happens when there are insufficient levels of dopamine in the brain – this is an important chemical for the proper movement of the body, thought processing and regulating moods.

Healthy fats, like those found in nuts and olive oil, plus the anti-inflammatory properties of the copious amounts of vegetables and fruits, are well known to help fight off age-related cognitive disorders. They help to counteract the harmful effects of exposure to free radicals and toxicity, food allergies and inflammation, all of which contribute towards an impairment in brain function. Studies show that people who adhere to the Mediterranean diet display lower rates of Alzheimer's than in any other diet. Adding probiotics, such as those found in kefir and yogurt, also help to promote a healthy gut, which, as we know, is vital for improving mood and memory disorders.

7. Can Help to Prolong Life Expectancy

Diets that are high in fresh plant-based foods and healthy fat have been shown to be the best combination for longevity. That main fat source in the Mediterranean diet is monounsaturated fat and is found in nuts and olive oil. Research over the years has shown that this is the best type of fat for lowering the risk of heart disease, depression, cancer, Alzheimer's disease, cognitive decline, inflammatory disease and much more besides. These diseases are the leading causes, in the developed nations, of death.

The Lyon Diet Heart Study looked at those who had suffered heart attacks between 1988 and 1992. The participants of the study were asked to either follow a Mediterranean type diet or follow a standard diet for the post-heart attack, which reduced saturated fat significantly. After 4 years, the results showed that those who followed the Mediterranean diet had 70% less heart disease, three times the risk-reduction that is achieved through statins, the prescription drug for lowering cholesterol. They also showed 45% less risk of all-cause death than those on the standard post-heart attack diet.

One thing that stood out among the results was that there was little change in levels of cholesterol which just shows that, contrary to what we are told, there is far more to heart disease than high cholesterol.

8. Helps you Relax

One last factor is that the Mediterranean diet encourages people to sleep better, spend more time in nature and bond with other people over a god healthy home-cooked meal. These are all great ways to lower stress levels, which, in turn, lowers inflammation. On the whole, people in the Mediterranean tend to spend more time outside and enjoy their meals with family and friends in a relaxed setting. They also set time aside to practice their hobbies, dance, laugh, enjoy the garden, and generally enjoy themselves.

Chapter 2: The Ten Commandments of the Mediterranean Diet

While we already know what the benefits of the Mediterranean diet are, actually adopting the proper Mediterranean way of eating is not quite as simple as you may believe, certainly not the way many cookbooks would have you believe. Yes, there are plenty of recipes that are promoted as being Mediterranean but they may not be the ones that are the best for us, according to the research. In many cases, these are dishes that are masquerading as the fare that we believe to be Mediterranean.

The main reason for this is because many cookery books seem to focus on desserts and festive foods from particular regions. We tend to think of foods like viros, souvlaki, and other meat-filled dishes but the real Mediterranean diet, the true one that was made famous back in the 1960's is more of a vegetarian based diet. It was called the "poor man's diet: because there wasn't much meat. More fish was included because it was more available but the main diet was legumes and plant foods, healthy sources of protein.

Casseroles were served which would contain little meat but plenty of vegetables such as peas, artichokes, carrots, and zucchini, and would always be accompanied by a side salad. On average a person would consume half a kilo each of vegetables and fruit per day.

To help you get the idea of what the diet actually involves, Dr. Catherine Itsopoulos, accredited practicing dietician, has come up with 10 commandments:

- Aim to consume around 60 ml of olive oil per day, using it as your main source of added fat
- Eat vegetables with every single meal, aiming for 100g of tomato, 100g of leafy greens and 200g of other vegetables per day.
- Eat at least two meals containing 250g of legumes each week
- Eat two servings of fish per week as a minimum guide. Each serving should be 150-200g and you should include oily fish, such as salmon, trevalla, sardines, mackerel, and gemfish. Canned tuna doesn't contain such high levels of omega-3 as tuna fillet, but is still a decent choice
- Eat meat, such as lamb, beef, pork, and chicken no more than a couple of times per week and make the portions small, bulking up with vegetables.
- Eat fresh fruit every single day and eat dried nuts and dried fruits for dessert or snacks
- Consume about 200g of yogurt every day and around 30-40g of cheese per day
- Make sure you include whole grain cereals and bread with your meals – aim for a consumption of about 3 or 4 slices of whole grain bread per day
- Drink red wine in moderation – a standard drink every day, about 100 ml. Only drink with meals and never over-indulge Try to keep away from alcohol entirely for two days of the week.
- Sweets and sugary drinks should only be consumed for special occasions and always in moderation.

Chapter 3: Busting the Mediterranean Diet Myths

There are plenty of benefits to the Mediterranean diet and no doubt you have heard loads of things about it. Not everything you read or hear is necessarily true, though, in particular, the claims that you can eat vast meals of rich food and knock back gallons of red wine. In this chapter, I am going to bust some of those myths that you may have heard about the Mediterranean diet:

1. Everyone who lies in the Mediterranean is healthy

The Mediterranean covers a vast amount of land and coast, including Greece, Turkey, Morocco, Italy, France, even parts of North Africa and not every region follows the same eating habits. For example, in northern Italy, they use more butter and lard in their cooking, consuming larger amounts of saturated fats, whereas, in southern Italy, they tend to use more olive oil. The basis for the Mediterranean diet for health is inspired by Greece, Crete, Morocco, southern Italy, and Spain.

2. You can eat vast amounts of cheese

Too much cheese does nothing more than pile on the pounds, high in calories and in saturated fat. While consumption of cheese is a Mediterranean practice, it is only in moderation and they tend to go for stronger cheeses, like goat cheese or feta. This can give you the flavor without eating a large amount of cheese.

3. Drinking copious amounts of red wine is good for your heart

While red wine does have health benefits, specifically for the heart, moderation is the real key. If you regularly drink more than a couple of glasses of wine, it can actually cause damage to your heart. One glass per day with a meal is the recommended amount for heart health.

4. It's fine to eat big portions of pasta with bread

Many people tend to think of Italian cooking, especially pasta when they think of the Mediterranean. Pasta needs bread otherwise you can't soak the sauce up. Yes, Italians do eat a lot of pasta but not in huge portions, the way Americans do. Mediterranean portions are typically side dishes and are around ½ to 1 cup. It is never served as a dish on its own and is generally accompanied by meat, salads, and vegetables. One slice of bread may also be consumed

5. You don't need to exercise on the Mediterranean diet

You do but you don't need to take out an expensive gym membership. The traditional Mediterranean lifestyle involves physical work and walking instead of driving. If you don't live a life where you can get out in the garden each day or walk instead of driving, then you will need to find alternative means of exercising every day.

6. Mediterranean people can eat huge meals and they never put on weight

This is technically not true. While Mediterranean people do tend to eat large meals, these are made up of several smaller dishes, usually low calorie, rather than one huge serving. They eat lots of raw and cooked vegetables, and small portions of legumes, meat, and grains. What is important is how the meal is made up, not how small or large it is. You can't eat whatever you want and expect to lose weight; it comes down to balance.

7. The Mediterranean diet is expensive
If you use legumes, beans and lentils as your main protein source and you stick to mainly whole grains and plants, the Mediterranean diet works out much cheaper than serving up processed and packaged foods.

8. The Mediterranean Diet is only based on food
While the food is a very big part of the Mediterranean diet, we must forget the other things that go into making up their way of life. When they eat, it isn't a rushed meal and it isn't in front of the TV; instead, they eat a leisurely meal with lots of company and this could be just as important as what you eat. Factor in the physical wok they do on a daily basis and the fact that they walk wherever they can, and you can see that this isn't just about the food.

9. All vegetable oils are good for you and they are all the same
If only things were that simple! There are actually two basic unsaturated vegetable oils – the traditional cold-pressed variety, such as peanut and extra-virgin olive oil that are high in healthy monounsaturated fats and made without heat or chemicals to extract the oils. The second are those that are processed in a modern way, like the sunflower, corn, soybean, cottonseed, canola, vegetable, and safflower oils. These are manufactured industrially from GM crops and use toxic solvents and high heat to get the oil out of the seeds. This kind of processing can damage the oil and turn the healthy fatty acids into trans fats, the most dangerous of all. They also contain a high level of omega-6, which upsets the omega 6 to 3 ratio that is vital for health.

Chapter 4: What You Should Be Eating (And What to Avoid)

There really isn't any right or wrong way to do the Mediterranean diet, simply because the Mediterranean is made up of so many countries that all eat differently. The basics of the diet for health are as follows but bear in mind that this is open to interpretation depending on your own circumstances, preferences, and needs.

What to Eat

Fish and Poultry

Eat two servings per week instead of red meat, which is limited to no more than 16 oz. a month.

- Turkey
- Chicken
- Shrimp
- Oysters
- Salmon
- Mackerel
- Squid
- Mussels
- Lobster
- Tuna
- Tilapia
- Founder
- Salmon

Healthy Fats

Stick to olive oil on the whole and canola on occasion. Olive oil is used as a seasoning and as a preparation food.

Vegetables and Fruits

Consume in abundance
- Artichokes
- Celery
- Eggplant
- Broccoli
- Peas
- Onions
- Peppers
- Lettuce
- Sweet potatoes
- Mushrooms
- Tomatoes
- Apples
- Melons
- Grapefruit
- Peaches
- Dates
- Strawberries
- Cherries
- Peaches

Dairy

Eat low to moderate amounts of milk, cheese, and yogurt but do use low or fat-free versions and try, where possible to eat those made by locally produced cow, sheep, and goat milk.

Grains

Eat whole grains only:

- wheat
- bulgar
- rice
- couscous
- barley
- spelt

Beverages
- One glass of red wine per day with a meal.
- Avoid sugary soft drinks, fruit juices, drink a little coffee and lots of water

Nuts

Eat in moderation and try to stick to nuts that grow on trees, like almonds, walnuts, and pecans. Choose unsalted nuts and do not eat those that have been candied

This list is clearly not exhaustive because there are so many different foods available across the Mediterranean. The rule of thumb is lots of fresh, local, and organic fruits and vegetables and where you eat dairy, meat or fish, opt for free range or wild-caught versions rather than those packaged in supermarkets

At all costs, avoid packaged and processed foods, sunflower and vegetable oils, margarine, anything with HCFS, added sugars and trans fats. Do read packet labels carefully

Just How Important is Olive Oil?

Virtually every nutritionist and researcher will attribute some of the health benefits of the diet to the generous amounts of olive oil that are used in every meal. Olives are, perhaps, one of the most ancient of foods, and olive trees have been growing across the Mediterranean since 3000 BC.

Olive oil is one of the elite foods containing healthy omega-3 fatty acids, joining the likes of walnuts and salmon. The health benefits of olive oil are firmly backed up by so much research that even the FDA has allowed the labels on bottles of olive oil to contain a health claim. Limited research, certainly not conclusive, suggests that consuming 2 tablespoons of olive oil every day is enough to cut the risk of heart disease because of the monounsaturated fat it contains. To achieve this, however, it is not enough to consume the olive oil; it has to be used to replace a similar level of saturated fat and not in addition to it.

So, what does olive oil, the mainstay of the Mediterranean diet, contain that makes it so good for you?

For a start, it is high in phenols, which are antioxidants that can fight damage caused by free radicals and lower inflammation. Olive oil is mainly monounsaturated fatty acids, with the most important of these being oleic acid. This is known to be healthy for the heart in several ways, especially when you compare it to hydrogenated, trans or refined fats and oils.

Olive oil is even a step above many of the grain-based carbohydrates when it comes to heart health. For example, the high levels of monounsaturated fats lower LDL cholesterol while raising HDL and reducing triglycerides far more effectively than a carb heavy diet does.

A beneficial amount of olive oil to consume on a daily basis is up to four tablespoons per day but this will depend on your caloric requirements. What you do have to remember is that there is more than one type of olive oil and this will have an effect. Many of the commercial manufacturers are trying to get on the olive oil health bandwagon by producing fake oil. These are nothing more than bad imitations that are actually bad for your health. The reason for this is because they are not harvested properly and are most certainly not processed in the right way and this can not only kill off some of the more delicate nutrients, it can also turn the fatty acids toxic or rancid.

To get the right oils, look for those that are labeled as cold-pressed and extra-virgin. Olive oil is, quite possibly, the most unique oil in that it can be consumed in its crude form without the need or any processing. You could actually press a bucket of olives and enjoy the oils as it comes.

One more tip about olive oil; if you are not sure if you have bought the real thing, put it in the freezer. True olive oil will NOT freeze so if it does its fake. Do make sure you purchase oil in dark glass bottles and do make sure the oil is made in the same region as the olives are harvested.

How to Follow the Mediterranean Diet at Restaurants

Most restaurant meals can be made suitable for the Mediterranean diet:

- Order seafood or fish for your main dish
- Ask them to use extra virgin olive oil for any fried foods
- Only consume whole grain bread and use olive oil rather than butter

Chapter 5: A Quick Start Guide to the Mediterranean Diet

Making the change is the hardest part about doing the Mediterranean diet but, to help you out, here are some simple guidelines and suggestions to help you get started:

- Swap vegetable oil for olive oil for sautéing
- Have a salad as a starter or side, have fruit as snacks and increase your vegetable intake
- Forget the refined pasta, bread, and rice; choose whole grain versions instead
- Cut red meat down by substituting 2 meals per week with fish
- Eat more dairy products, such as cheese, milk, and yogurt. Go for plain yogurt that you can dress up with nuts, fruit, and honey. Enjoy natural cheeses made from sheep, cow, and goat milk, locally produced. Whole milk products are linked to lower levels of body fat and a lower risk of obesity, mostly because these products make you feel fuller for longer.
- Eat more vegetables. Try eating a plate of tomatoes sliced up with olive oil and feta cheese. Layer peppers and mushrooms on your pizza instead of pepperoni and sausage. Eat more salad, homemade soups, and platters of crudités to get more vegetables into your diet
- You must change how you see meat – it is not a big part of the diet and, where you do eat it, you should opt for the grass-fed versions instead of that which has been industrially raised. Add strips of organic chicken to a salad and add a little amount of meat to a whole-wheat pasta dish

- Never miss breakfast. Start the day the right way with whole grains, fruit and any other food rich in fiber that keeps you satiated for longer
- Make sure you eat a seafood dish twice a week. The best ones, those rich in omega-3 fatty acids, are the salmon, tuna, black cod, herring, sardines, oysters, mussels, and clams.
- Have a vegetarian meal once a week, building your meal up around vegetables, whole grains, and beans. When you get used to it, increase to twice a week.
- Always use the good fats in your meals. Go for the extra virgin olive oil, avocado, olives and sunflower seeds as well as nuts in moderation
- If you have a sweet tooth, swap the cakes and ice cream for fresh fruit like fresh figs with honey, strawberries, apples and grapes, all locally grown produce.

Mercury in Fish

We all know that fish has massive health benefits but there are also the concerns over pollutants, such as traces of the mercury, a toxic heavy metal. This is found in just about all fish and shellfish and you need to be able to make the right and the safest choices when you buy fish.

The rule of thumb is that, the larger the fish, the higher the concentration of pollutants and mercury. Try to avoid the largest fish, such as king mackerel, shark, tilefish, and swordfish.

You should be able to safely consume around 12 oz. of cooked seafood per week, split into 2 portions of 6 oz. each

If you are eating locally caught seafood, pay attention to any advisories about what is safe to eat and what you should avoid

If you are pregnant or nursing a child, or are a child under the age of 12, go for fish that have the lower levels of mercury, such as canned light tuna, shrimp, pollock, salmon, and catfish. If you eat Albacore tuna, be aware that it has a higher level of mercury and, as such, you should eat no more than 6 oz. per week

Ideas for Alternative Foods

You should start slowly, swapping foods out gradually to get yourself used to the Mediterranean diet. Try these delicious food swaps:

Instead of:	Try This:
Pretzels, chips, crackers with ranch dip celery, carrots with salsa	Broccoli,
White rice and a stir-fried meat some stir-fried vegetables	Quinoa with
Sandwiches made with white bread/rolls fillings in whole-wheat tortillas	Healthy
Ice cream made with milk	Puddings
Toast for breakfast with fruit and honey	Plain yogurt

Now that you know the basics of the Mediterranean diet, it's time to look at some recipes so that you can see just how satisfying the diet is.

Chapter 6: Breakfast

Yogurt with Honey and Apricots

Preparation time: 5 minutes
Serves 6

Ingredients
- 1 cup of Greek yogurt, low fat
- 2 tbsp. organic honey
- ½ tsp vanilla extract
- 9 fresh apricots, cut in half lengthways

Instructions
1. Whisk the yogurt together with the vanilla and honey
2. Arrange the apricots in bowls and spoon the yogurt mixture over the top
3. Serve straight away or chill first

Mediterranean Stuffed Tomatoes

Preparation time: 10 minutes
Cooking time: 5 minutes
Serves 1

Ingredients:

- 2 large tomatoes
- ½ cup garlic croutons, pre-packaged or homemade
- ¼ cup goat cheese, crumbled
- ¼ cup Kalamata olives, pitted and sliced
- 2 tbsp. Italian salad dressing or low fat vinaigrette
- 2 tbsp. fresh chopped basil or thyme

Instructions:

1. Preheat the broiler
2. Slice the tomatoes in half crossways
3. Discard the seeds, using your finger to push them out
4. Use a small knife to remove the pulp – you should be left with two shells
5. Chop up the pulp and put it into a medium bowl
6. Put the tomato shells onto a paper towel, cut side down and leave to drain for 5 minutes
7. Add the olives, croutons, goats cheese and herbs in the bowl with the tomato pulp and mix together; add the dressing and combine well
8. Spoon the mixture into the hollowed-out tomato shells
9. Place them on a baking tray or a broiler pan and broil for about 5 minutes. They should be 4 or 5 inches away from the heat and the cheese should be melted
10. Serve straightaway

Breakfast Couscous

Preparation time: 20 minutes
Cooking time: 5 minutes
Serves 4

Ingredients:
- 3 cups low fat milk, 1%
- 1 cinnamon stick, about 2 inches in length
- 1 cup whole wheat couscous, uncooked
- ¼ cup dried currants
- ½ cup dried chopped apricots
- 6 tsp dark brown soft sugar
- ¼ tsp salt
- 4 tsp melted butter

Instructions:
1. Place the milk into a large pan and heat with the cinnamon stick for 3 minutes over a medium-high heat. Do not allow to boil, just let bubbles begin to form around the edge of the milk
2. Take the milk from the heat and add the couscous, fruit, salt, and 4 tsp of sugar. Mix together well and cover; leave to stand for 15 minutes
3. Take the cinnamon stick out and divide the mixture between 4 bowls
4. Top off with 1 tsp of melted butter and ½ tsp sugar' serve straightaway

Greek Yogurt with Honey, Oats, and Mixed Berries

Preparation time: 5 minutes
Serves 1

Ingredients:
- ¼ Greek yogurt, full fat
- ¼ cup fresh or frozen mixed berries
- ¼ cup oats
- Small handful of fresh walnuts
- Honey

Instructions:
1. Put the berries into a bowl. If they are frozen, microwave for 30 seconds
2. Add the yogurt, walnuts, and oats
3. Mix gently and drizzle honey over the top
4. Serve straightaway or chill first

Avocado Toast

Preparation time: 5 minutes
Cooking time: 5 minutes
Serves 2

Ingredients:
- 2 avocados, small and ripe, pitted, and peeled
- ¾ cup crumbled feta cheese
- 2 tbsp. fresh chopped mint, plus a little extra for garnishing
- 4 slices wholegrain rye bread
- Squeeze of lemon juice

Instructions:
1. Roughly mash the avocado with a fork in a medium bowl
2. Add the mint and mix in with a squeeze of lemon juice, mashing until combined
3. Season with salt and pepper
4. Toast the bread and spoon the avocado mixture over the toast
5. Top off with feta and serve with a garnish of fresh mint

For a larger meal, add some shaved ham or a poached egg

Frittata

Preparation time: 10 minutes
Cooking time 25 minutes
Serves 6

Ingredients:
- 1 cup chopped onion
- 2 cloves minced garlic
- 3 tbsp. extra virgin olive oil
- 8 beaten eggs
- ¼ cup light cream, milk or half and half
- ½ cup feta, crumbled
- ½ cup bottled roasted red pepper, chopped
- ½ cup Kalamata or other olives, pitted
- ¼ cup fresh slivered basil
- 1/8 tsp ground black pepper
- ½ cup garlic and onion croutons, crushed coarsely
- 2 tbsp. parmesan cheese, shredded finely
- Fresh basil leaves for garnish

Instructions:
1. Preheat your broiler
2. In a broiler-proof pan or skillet, heat the oil and cook the garlic and onion for about 2 minutes, or until the onion is tender
3. Mix the beaten eggs with the milk in a separate bowl
4. Stir in the peppers, feta, olives, black pepper, and basil
5. Pour the mixture over the onions and cook until set, running a spatula around the edge to lift the mixture as it sets. This ensures that all the mixture is cooked
6. Mix the croutons with 1 tbsp. oil. And the cheese and sprinkle it over the frittata mixture

7. Broil about 4 inches away from the heat until the crumbs have turned golden and the top is set firmly
8. Cut into wedges and serve with fresh basil leaves

Chapter 7: Soups

Fish Soup

Preparation time: 15 minutes
Cooking time: 30 minutes
Serves 4

Ingredients:

- 1 lb. live mussels
- 1 lb. live clams
- 1 lb. white fish cut into ½ inch slices – Monkfish is a good one
- 1 lb. uncooked prawns or shrimps with shells on
- 4 small calamari (squid)
- 4 finely chopped garlic cloves
- ½ liter fish stock OR one fish stock cube
- 8 ½ oz dry white wine
- 1 small red pepper, roasted and diced finely
- Juice from ½ a lemon
- 1 bunch chopped parsley
- 1 tsp turmeric powder
- 1 tsp corn flour or corn starch
- Salt and pepper for seasoning

Instructions:

1. Put the wine and stock into a large pan and heat; add the mussels and cook until they open. Remove any that don't open and if you don't use all of the mussels, freeze them on the half shell
2. Remove the opened mussels and add the clams to the liquid
3. Cook until they open, discarding any that don't

35

4. Remove the clams and add shrimp or prawns to the liquid, cooking until pink. These are for garnish so don't use too many

5. Remove the cooked prawns and set aside

6. Shell the remainder of the prawns

7. Slice the squid into ½ inch rounds and fry the squid and prawns in olive oil with the garlic until cooked through

8. Strain the liquid using a fine sieve and return it to the pan

9. Add the white fish and cook over a medium heat, stirring until cooked

10. Add the turmeric, lemon juice, corn flour and most of the parsley; bring back to a simmer

11. Add the clams, shrimp, and squid back to the liquid and heat through

12. Arrange the mussels and the first lot of prawns on soup plates and pour the soup over the top

13. Sprinkle the rest of the parsley over the top and serve hot

Tomato Soup

Preparation time: 10 minutes
Cooking time: 15 minutes
Serves 4

Ingredients:
The Soup

- 2 cans Italian plum tomatoes, chopped (16 oz. cans) OR use the same weight of fresh skinned and chopped tomatoes
- 32 oz. vegetable stock
- 1 tsp tomato puree
- 1 rough chopped medium onion
- 2 bashed garlic cloves
- 1 tsp sugar
- 1 tsp dried basil
- Small handful fresh basil leaves
- Half a lemon, juiced
- 4 oz. Greek yogurt
- Salt and pepper for seasoning

The Croutons

1. 12 thin slices of a stale baguette, whole meal
2. Olive oil
3. 1 oz. parmesan cheese, fresh grated

Instructions:

1. Heat a little olive oil and sauté the onion; do not let it brown
2. Add the garlic, turn down the heat and sauté for a few minutes

3. Add the basil, tomato, sugar, and the stock and bring up to the boil
4. While it cooks, sprinkle the bread slices with olive oil and top off with the grated cheese; grill until golden
5. Allow the soup to boil gently for a minute or 2 and then use a stick blender to blend it in the pan
6. Spoon into bowls and stop off with the croutons and fresh basil leaves

Sweet Potato Soup

Preparation time: 10 minutes
Cooking time: 40 minutes
Serves 4-6

Instructions:

- 2 tbsp. extra virgin olive oil
- 1 large chopped onion
- 2 lb. sweet potato, peeled and chopped into medium size pieces
- ½ tsp ground cumin
- ¼ tsp ground chili
- ¼ tsp ground cinnamon
- ½ tsp ground coriander
- ¼ tsp salt
- A little more than 2 cups chicken stock
- Low fat crème Fraiche for garnish
- Fresh chopped coriander or parsley for garnish

Instructions:

1. Heat the olive oil over a high heat and sauté the onion until it begins to color
2. Turn the heat to medium and sauté the garlic for a few minutes, stirring well
3. Add the sweet potato to the pan and sauté for a few minutes
4. Add the spices and salt, stir well, and cook for 2 minutes
5. Pour the stock in, increase the heat and bring up to the boil; give it one more stir and cover the pan
6. Reduce the heat and simmer for 2 minutes until the potato has softened

7. Take the pan off the heat and use a hand blender to blend until smooth
8. If the soup is too thick, add a little stock or water
9. Season to taste and serve in warm bowls.
10. Swirl the crème Fraiche through the soup and garnish with the parsley or coriander

Seafood Bisque

Preparation time: 20 minutes
Cooking time: 60 minutes
Serves 4

Ingredients:
The Soup
- 1 lb. uncooked, shell-on shrimp or prawns – peeled and heads removed (reserve for the stock)
- 8 oz. white fish, chopped into cubes
- 1 chopped small onion
- 1 chopped leek
- 1 stalk chopped celery
- 1 peeled and chopped carrot
- 1 large garlic clove, chopped
- 1 carton single cream, 100 ml
- Olive oil
- Juice from ½ lemon

The Stock
1. 1 peeled onion, chopped into quarters
2. 1 rough chopped carrot
3. 12 black peppercorns
4. 1 tsp fennel seed
5. 1 tsp turmeric powder
6. ½ bottle white wine, medium sweet and an equal amount of water
7. Small handful parsley, rough chopped
8. Prawn shells and heads
9. 2 whole cloves
10. 4 bashed garlic cloves
11. 2 whole bay leaves
12. Juice from ½ lemon

The Croutons
- 1 small whole meal baguette, sliced thinly
- Olive oil
- ½ tsp Herbes de Provence

Instructions:
1. Peel the prawns and leave to one side
2. Make the stock by putting all of the stock ingredients into a large pan and bringing up to the boil
3. Leave to simmer for about 15 minutes, on occasion crushing the prawn heads and shells with a wooden spoon
4. Strain the stock and discard all of the solid bits
5. Poach 4 prawns lightly in the stock until they are just cooked and then remove them, leaving them to one side for garnish
6. Fry the carrot, onion, leek, and celery in some olive oil until they are soft, around 10 minutes
7. Turn the heat down and add the garlic cook for about 5 minutes
8. Add the stock and bring up to the boil
9. Add the white fish and prawns and poach for about 3 minutes
10. Remove the stock from the heat and blend it until smooth with a stick blender
11. Add the cream and season to taste
12. If serving now, keep it warm; if not cool it and refrigerate
13. Now make the croutons by frying the baguette slices in the oil until golden; drain on paper towels and sprinkle the herbs over the top
14. Serve the warm soup garnished with a prawn and a little smoked paprika and the croutons

Cauliflower Soup

Preparation time: 10 minutes
Cooking time: 30 minutes
Serves 4

Ingredients:
- Extra virgin olive oil for sautéing
- 2 large leeks, sliced finely
- 3 large celery stalks, sliced thinly
- 2 bashed garlic cloves
- 1 heaped tsp ground cumin
- 1 level tsp turmeric powder
- 1 small dried ground chili (optional)
- 1 lb. chopped cauliflower florets
- 1 medium peeled and diced potato
- 1 liter vegetable stock
- Salt and pepper for seasoning

Instructions:
1. Heat a little oil and sauté the celery and leek until soft and golden
2. Add the garlic and turn the heat down; sauté for a minute or 2, stirring
3. Add the turmeric, cumin, and the chili if using it and sauté gently, stirring, for about 1 minute
4. Add the potato and cauliflower, pour in the stock and stir
5. Season and bring to the boil; cover and simmer for 10 minutes or so, until the cauliflower and potato are cooked. Remove from the heat
6. Blend roughly with a hand blender, leaving some of the vegetable chunks whole
7. Season to tastes and serve with croutons or on its own

White Bean Soup

Preparation time: 20 minutes
Cooking time: 30 minutes
Serves 4

Ingredients:
- 1 tbsp. vegetable oil
- 1 chopped onion
- 1 chopped celery stalk
- 1 minced garlic clove
- 2 cans, 16 oz. each, white kidney beans
- 1 14 oz. can chicken broth
- ¼ tsp ground black pepper
- 1/8 tsp dried thyme
- 2 cups water
- 1 bunch fresh washed and sliced spinach
- 1 tbsp. freshly squeezed lemon juice

Instructions:
1. Heat the oil in a large pan and cook the celery and onion for about 5 to 8 minutes, or until they are soft
2. Add the garlic and cook for a further 30 seconds, stirring continually
3. Drain and rinse the beans and stir in, adding the broth, thyme, pepper, and water
4. Bring up to a boil, turn the heat down and simmer for about 15 minutes
5. Remove 2 cups of the vegetables from the soup, using a slotted spoon and set to one side
6. Blend the rest of the soup on a low speed until smooth – do it in batches if necessary

7. Pour the soup back into the pan and stir the reserved vegetables back in
8. Bring up to a boil, stirring occasionally, and then add the spinach, cooking for about a minute until the spinach has wilted
9. Stir the lemon juice in, and serve with a garnish of grated parmesan cheese

Chapter 8: Salads

Fennel Tuna and Egg Salad with Olives

Preparation time: 15 minutes
Cooking time: 5 – 10 minutes
Serves 4

Ingredients:
The Dressing:
- 1 tsp fresh lemon zest
- 1 tbsp. fresh lemon juice
- 4 tbsp. extra virgin olive oil
- 1 tsp fennel greens, chopped
- ¼ tsp salt
- Salt and pepper for seasoning

The Salad:
- 1 small peeled red onion, sliced into thin rounds
- Rice or white wine vinegar
- 1 yellow seeded pepper, veins removed and sliced thinly
- 2 small fennel bulbs, trimmed and sliced lengthways, thinly
- 8 radishes, French Breakfast variety if possible
- 12 green and black olives
- 2 hardboiled eggs, sliced into quarters
- 1 small can of tuna in water, drained
- 1 tbsp. capers

Instructions:
1. To make the dressing, combine the juice, zest, salt, oil, and ground pepper in a bowl; stir the fennel greens in

2. To make the salad, toss the slices of onion in some vinegar and leave to marinate. Turn them occasionally so that they are brightly colored.

3. Arrange the rings of pepper on a plate and top off with the fennel slices

4. Alternate the olives and radishes around the edge of the platter and place the tuna into the middle

5. Scatter the tuna with capers and arrange the egg quarters around the edge of it

6. Drain the onion and arrange over the salad

7. Spoon dressing over and serve

Greek Salad Skewers

Preparation time: 20 minutes
Cooking time: 5 minutes
Serves 4

Ingredients:
- 2 oz. cubed feta
- 2 tbsp. extra virgin olive oil
- ½ tsp dried oregano
- 1 lemon, sliced into 6 wedges
- 2 slices Italian bread, 1 inch thick and cut into 16 cubes of 1 inch
- 16 cherry tomatoes
- 1 can artichoke hearts, drained and cut in half lengthways (14 oz. can)
- ½ small red onion, peeled and chopped into 1 inch cubes
- 1 small sliced cucumber
- 20 leaves of romaine lettuce (inner leaves only)
- 12 olives, assorted, pitted

Instructions:
1. Soak 8 bamboo skewers, about 8-10 inches in water for half an hour
2. Toss the feta in oregano and oil and squeeze two of the lemon wedges over the top. Season to taste
3. Lightly oil a grill
4. Thread each bamboo skewer with alternate chunks of bread, artichoke, tomato, and onion
5. Coat with a little olive oil and grill until golden brown, turning to cook all over, about 4 minutes – do remove before the tomato falls apart.

6. Arrange the lettuce between 4 plates and top off with 2 skewers on each plate
7. Divide the feta mix between the plates
8. Divide the cucumber and olives between each plate and serve garnished with a wedge of lemon

Potato Salad, Mediterranean-Style

Preparation time: 10 minutes
Cooking time: 35-45 minutes
Serves 4

Ingredients:
- 1 tbsp. extra virgin olive oil
- 1 small thinly sliced onion
- 1 crushed garlic clove
- 1 tsp fresh or dried oregano
- ½ lb. cherry tomatoes, canned
- ¼ lb. sliced roast red pepper from a jar
- ¾ lb. new potato, sliced in half if a large one
- 3/4 oz. sliced black olives
- Handful torn fresh basil leaves

Instructions:
1. Heat the oil in a large pan and cook the onion for about 5 or 10 minutes, until softened
2. Add the oregano and the garlic and cook for a further minute
3. Add the peppers and tomatoes, season, and simmer for about 10 minutes
4. Cook the potato in salted boiling water until tender, about 10 or 15 minutes
5. Drain and mix with the sauce
6. Serve warm sprinkled with basil and olives

Fig and Mozzarella Salad

Preparation time: 5 minutes
Cooking time: 5 minutes
Serves 2

Ingredients:
- ½ lb. trimmed green beans
- 6 small fresh figs, cut into quarters
- 1 thin sliced shallot
- 1 ball of mozzarella, about 4 ½ oz., drained and torn into chunks
- 1 ¾ oz. toasted and chopped hazelnuts
- Small handful of torn fresh basil leaves
- 3 tbsp. balsamic vinegar
- 1 tbsp. fig relish or jam
- 3 tbsp. extra virgin olive oil

Instructions:
1. Blanch the beans in boiling salted water for about 2 or 3 minutes
2. Drain and rinse in cold water and drain again on kitchen paper
3. Arrange the beans on a plate and top off with the shallot, figs, hazelnuts, mozzarella, and basil
4. Put the fig jam, vinegar, and olive oil into a small-lidded jar, season, and seal. Shake well and drizzle over the salad before serving

Feta and Watermelon Salad with Fresh Crisp bread

Preparation time: 70 minutes
Cooking time: 1 hour
Serves 4

Ingredients:
The Salad
- ½ a fresh watermelon (1 ½ kg), deseeded, peeled and chopped into chunks
- ½ lb. feta cheese, cut into cubes
- A large handful of pitted black olives
- A handful of fresh flat-leaf parsley and mint leaves chopped roughly
- 1 red onion, finely sliced in rings
- Balsamic vinegar and olive oil for serving

The Crisp bread
- ½ lb. bread mix, white
- 1 tbsp. extra virgin olive oil, plus extra
- Plain flour for dusting
- 1 beaten egg white
- Fennel, poppy, and sesame seed for scattering

Instructions:
1. Make the bread mix by following the pack instructions and include 1 tbsp. olive oil in it
2. Leave it in a warm place for 1 hour to rise until it is double the size
3. In the meantime, preheat your oven to 220° F
4. Divide the risen dough into 6 equal pieces and roll out on a floured surface, as thin as possible

5. Transfer the flat dough to baking trays and brush with the beaten egg white and scatter the seeds over the top
6. Bake until brown and crisp, about 15 minutes
7. You can do this the day before if you want and store them in an airtight container until you need them
8. Toss the melon with the olives and feta and scatter the onion and herbs over the top
9. Serve on plates and drizzle the vinegar and oil over the top
10. Serve with the crisp breads

Tuscan Tuna Salad

Preparation time: 10 minutes
Serves 4

Ingredients:
- 2 cans tuna in water or oil, drained (6 oz. cans)
- 10 cherry tomatoes, cut into quarters
- 4 trimmed and sliced scallions
- 2 tbsp. extra virgin olive oil
- 2 tbsp. freshly squeezed lemon juice
- ¼ tsp salt
- 1 15 oz. can white beans, drained and rinsed
- Ground black pepper for seasoning

Instructions:
1. Mix the beans, tuna, scallions, tomatoes, lemon juice, pepper, oil, and salt together gently
2. Refrigerate until ready to use

Chapter 9: Main Courses

Tomato and Eggplant Pasta Bake

Preparation time: 15 minutes
Cooking time: 40 minutes
Serves 6

Ingredients:
- 1 lb. eggplant, cubed
- 1 lb. small tomatoes, about 2 inches in diameter, cut in half
- 1 large bell pepper, red, chopped coarsely
- 1 large onion, chopped coarsely
- 8 oz. quinoa rotelle OR whole wheat fusilli
- ¼ cup fresh basil pesto
- 4 tbsp. fresh basil, chopped
- ¼ cup parmesan, finely grated
- ¼ tsp salt
- ¼ tsp ground black pepper

Instructions:
1. Heat your broiler
2. Place the tomatoes, cut-side up, on an oiled baking tray with the eggplant, onion, and bell pepper.
3. Coat the vegetables with a little olive oil and season with the salt and pepper
4. Broil until the vegetables are tender and golden brown in color, stirring al except for the tomatoes.
5. In the meantime, heat your oven to 375° F
6. Cook the pasta as per the package instructions
7. Drain well and toss with the vegetables, the pesto and half of the fresh chopped basil

8. Spoon into an oiled shallow baking pan and top off with the cheese
9. Cover the pan with foil and bake until warmed through, about 15 or 20 minutes
10. Serve sprinkled with the rest of the fresh basil

Whole Roasted Fish with Lemon and Oregano

Preparation time: 20 minutes
Cooking time: 20 minutes
Serves 4

Ingredients:
- 1 tbsp. extra virgin olive oil
- 2 tsp freshly squeezed lemon juice
- ½ tsp dried oregano
- 1 tsp salt
- ¼ tsp ground black pepper
- 2 sliced garlic cloves
- 2 whole sea bass, cleaned
- 8 slices of lemon

Instructions:
1. Preheat your broiler or grill and oil the rack lightly
2. Whisk the oil with the juice, pepper, oregano, and half of the salt; set to one side
3. Make 3 vertical shallow slits on each side of both fish
4. Rub the rest of the salt into the fish
5. Brush the oil mixture on the inside of the fish; stuff the garlic and lemon slices inside the fish
6. Grill for about 15 to 20 minutes, turning twice and basting with the rest of the oil mixture until the fish is a golden-brown color and the flesh has started turning opaque
7. Leave it to rest for about 10 minutes before you serve with a side salad

Greek Chicken

Preparation time: 2 hours
Cooking time: 6 minutes
Serves 4

Ingredients:
The Chicken
- 4 chicken breast halves, skinless and boneless
- 1 tbsp. freshly squeezed lemon juice
- 1 tbsp. extra virgin olive oil
- ½ tsp salt
- ¼ tsp ground black pepper
- 1 tsp dried oregano
- 1 minced garlic clove

The Yogurt
- 1 ¼ cup fat-free Greek yogurt
- ½ cup shredded cucumber
- 2 minced cloves garlic
- 1 tsp freshly chopped dill
- ½ cup pistachios, shelled and chopped coarsely

Instructions:
1. Butterfly the chicken breast. To do this, place a breast piece on a surface, shiny side facing up and with the pointed end facing you. Put your hand on the chicken breast and, holding a knife in a parallel position to the table, push it into the thickest part of the chicken and slice almost through the chicken. Open it up like a book and gently flatten it. Repeat with the rest of the chicken

2. Mix the oil, oregano, lemon juice and garlic together and marinade the chicken in it for a couple of hours in the refrigerator. Turn the chicken occasionally
3. Put the yogurt into a coffee strainer set over a bowl and refrigerate for up to 2 hours to drain
4. Mix the yogurt with the dill, cucumber, garlic, and half of the pistachios
5. Preheat the grill
6. Take the chicken out of the marinade and sprinkle the salt and pepper over
7. Grill on an oiled grill rack for a couple of minutes on each side until cooked all the way through
8. Serve the chicken topped off with the yogurt and garnished with the rest of the pistachios

Barley Risotto with Mushrooms

Preparation time: 15 minutes
Cooking time: 35 minutes
Serves 6

Ingredients:
- 1 oz. dried mushroom
- 2 cups boiling water
- 2 cups low salt beef broth
- 2 tsp extra virgin olive oil
- 1/4 lb. sliced button mushrooms
- 1 small chopped onions
- 3 chopped garlic cloves
- 1 cup barley
- 2 tsp dried sage
- ¼ tsp salt
- ½ cup parmesan cheese, grated

Instructions:
1. Mix the dried mushrooms with the boiling water and leave it to stand for about 15 minutes
2. Place a coffee filter or some paper towels into a fine sieve and set it over a saucepan
3. Pour the steeped mushrooms through the sieve, retaining the liquid
4. Chop the mushrooms and leave to one side
5. Add the broth to the mushroom liquid and heat over a medium heat
6. Warm up the oil in a Dutch oven on a medium heat and cook all of the mushrooms, garlic, and onion for a few minutes, stirring occasionally

7. Add the sage, barley, and salt, stir, and cook for 2 minutes
8. Add a cup of the broth and cook for 5 minutes, stirring constantly – the broth should be absorbed into the mixture
9. Continue cooking and stirring for about 20 or 25 minutes, adding the broth ½ cup at a time, until the barley is tender and the liquid is absorbed
10. Serve topped with the cheese

Lemon-Turkey Cutlets

Preparation time: 10 minutes
Cooking time: 20 minutes
Serves 4

Ingredients:

- ¼ cup all-purpose flour
- 1 large egg
- 4 turkey breast cutlets, skinless and boneless, cut in half crossways
- 2 tbsp. extra virgin olive oil
- ½ lemon sliced into 8 thin slices
- 2 tbsp. pitted green olives or capers, rinsed, drained and chopped
- ½ cup dry white wine
- 1 cup low salt chicken broth
- 1 tbsp. butter unsalted variety
- ¼ tsp salt
- ¼ tsp ground black pepper
- ¼ cup flat leaf parsley, chopped – optional

Instructions:

1. Mix the flour with the salt and pepper on a shallow plate
2. Add 1 tbsp. water to the egg and beat well in a shallow bowl
3. Dredge the turkey pieces in the flour and shake the excess off
4. Dip in the egg, coating thoroughly and drip the excess off
5. Heat the oil in a large pan on a medium high heat

6. Cook the turkey for about 6 or 7 minutes, turning, until cooked through and golden brown
7. Remove the turkey from the pan and leave to one side
8. Cook the capers/olives and lemon slices in the pan until the lemon has gone a golden-brown color, around 2 minutes
9. Remove the lemon and set aside
10. Add the wine to the pan, follow with the broth and simmer for about 6 minutes, until it has thickened a little
11. Put the turkey back in the pan and stir the parsley and butter in
12. Simmer for about 5 minutes, or until the turkey is warmed through
13. Serve with the lemon slices

Scallops Provençale

Preparation time: 35 minutes
Cooking time: 50 minutes
Serves 8

Ingredients:

- 2 tbsp. unsalted butter
- 1 lb. rinsed and drained sea scallops
- 1 small finely chopped onion
- ½ lb. thin sliced mushrooms
- 1 minced garlic clove
- 2 peeled and chopped medium tomatoes
- ¼ cup dry white wine
- 2 tbsp. ketchup
- ½ tsp salt
- ½ tsp dried and chopped tarragon
- ¼ tsp dried rosemary
- Pinch of white pepper
- ¼ lb. small cooked shrimp, frozen
- 2 tsp white wine vinegar
- Fresh chopped parsley for garnish

Instructions:

1. Preheat your oven to 400° F
2. Heat the butter over a medium heat and lightly brown off the scallops – don't crowd them, cook in batches if necessary. Remove the scallops and place them in buttered baking shells or individual casserole dishes
3. Cook the mushrooms and onions in the skillet until the onion softens and starts to brown
4. Stir the tomatoes, garlic, and ketchup. Wine, salt, herbs, and white pepper in, and bring to a boil

5. Cover the pan, turn the heat down and simmer for about 15 minutes
6. Uncover and cook for a further 3 minutes or until it has thickened
7. Mix the vinegar and shrimp in and then spoon the mixture over the scallops
8. Bake until the sauce has started to bubble and has begun to brown around the edges, around 10 minutes
9. Serve garnished with parsley

Chapter 10: Desserts

Baklava

Preparation time: 20 minutes
Cooking time: 35 minutes
Makes 24 pieces

Ingredients:
- 3 cups coarsely chopped unsalted pistachio nuts
- 1/3 cup sugar
- 2 tsp fresh orange zest
- ¼ tsp ground cloves
- 1/8 tsp unsalted butter
- Cooking spray – butter flavored if you can get it
- 24 sheets phyllo pastry, 17 by 12 inch, cut in half crossways
- 1 tbsp. water
- ¾ cup organic honey
- ¼ cup fresh squeezed orange juice
- 1 tbsp. freshly squeezed lemon juice
- ½ tsp ground cardamom

Instructions:
1. Preheat your oven to 350° F
2. Put the pistachios in a bowl with the orange zest, sugar, salt, and cloves; combine well and set to one side
3. Oil a 9 by 13-inch baking dish with the spray
4. Place one sheet of phyllo length ways in the base of the dish and drape one end over the end of the dish
5. Spray lightly with cooking spray
6. Repeat with 5 more sheets

7. Sprinkle 1/3 of the nut mixture over the top
8. Repeat this procedure twice more
9. With the last nut layer, coat with 6 phyllo sheets, oiled and then oil the top sheet, pressing it down gently into the dish
10. Sprinkle a little water over the top
11. Make 6 even crossways cuts and 4 even lengthways cuts to make 24 portions
12. Bake for 30 minutes until golden brown
13. In the meanwhile, mix the lemon and orange juice, the honey, and the cardamom together over a low heat and cook for about 2 minutes or until the honey has dissolved completely
14. Drizzle over the baklava and leave to cool off completely before serving

Baked Apple

Preparation time: 10 minutes
Cooking time: 45 minutes
Serves 2

Ingredients:
- 2 large cooking apples, sharp rather than sweet
- 2 tbsp. organic honey
- ¼ tsp ground cinnamon
- ¼ tsp mixed spice
- 1 ½ oz. walnuts, roughly chopped
- 1 ½ oz. sultanas, roughly chopped
- Juice and zest of ½ lemon

Instructions:
1. Preheat your oven to 350° F
2. Use a corer or a sharp knife to remove the cores from the apples
3. Around the center of each apple, make a continuous cut, about 1/8-inch deep
4. Cut a little piece of apple from the core and push it down the center of the apple, sealing the hole at the base
5. Put both apples into a baking dish
6. Mix all the other ingredients together, combining thoroughly
7. Divide the mixture between the two apples, pushing it down firmly into the center of them and finishing with a small mound on the top
8. Pour ½ inch of water into the dish
9. Bake for about 40 or 45 minutes in the center of the oven, until the apple is golden brown and soft
10. Serve straightaway, pouring the juice over the top and adding a little crème Fraiche

Lemon Pudding

Preparation time: 5 minutes
Cooking time: 5 minutes
Serves 4

Ingredients:
- ¾ cup sugar
- ¼ cup cornstarch
- 2 ½ cups milk
- 3 egg yolks, beaten lightly
- Zest from 2 lemons
- A pinch of salt
- Juice from 2 lemons
- 2 tsp butter, unsalted
- Crushed digestive biscuits and whipped cream for decorating

Instructions:
1. Whisk the cornstarch and the sugar together
2. Add in the milk and whisk until you have a smooth consistency
3. Now whisk the salt, zest, and egg yolks in, combining thoroughly
4. Pour the mixture into a pan and heat over a medium heat, stirring constantly with a wooden spoon until the sauce is thick enough to coat the back of a spoon
5. Take the pan off the heat and stir the butter and lemon juice in
6. Divide the mixture between 4 bowls and leave to cool before covering with plastic wrap and chilling for several hours
7. Before you serve, sprinkle with crushed biscuit and whipped cream

Orange and Lemon Ricotta Cake

Preparation time: 15 minutes
Cooking time: 70 minutes
Serves 8

Ingredients:

- 3 lb. fresh ricotta cheese
- 8 whole eggs
- ½ lb. sugar
- Zest from a fresh orange
- Zest from a fresh lemon
- Butter to coat the pan

Instructions:

1. Preheat the oven to 425° F
2. Mix all of the ingredients together thoroughly in a bowl
3. Coat a 9-inch pan all over with butter
4. Pour in the mixture, coating the pan evenly
5. Bake for 30 minutes
6. Reduce the heat to 380° F and cook for a further 40 minutes
7. Cool before serving

Pavlova

Preparation time: 15 minutes
Cooking time: 3 hours
Serves 4

Ingredients:

- 7 oz. castor sugar
- 4 egg whites
- 2 tsp vinegar
- 1 tbsp. corn starch or corn flour
- 1 cup whipping cream
- 1 segmented orange
- 1 sliced kiwi
- 6 or 8 large ripe strawberries

Instructions:

1. Preheat the oven to 300° F
2. Whisk up the egg whites until stiff peaks are formed
3. Whisk the sugar in, one tbsp. at a time and then whisk in the vinegar
4. Lastly, whisk in the cornstarch
5. Line a flat baking tray with baking paper and grease it with olive oil spray
6. Put the meringue mix onto the paper in a 10-inch circle. It should be 3 ½ inches deep
7. Put the meringue into the middle of the oven, shut the door and immediately reduce the heat to 245° F
8. Cook for about 2 ½ to 3 hours until the meringue is a creamy color and crisp to touch
9. Turn off the oven and leave the meringue to cool down totally
10. When cold, peel the greaseproof paper off

11. Place the pavlova on a plate and pile on thickly whipped cream, spreading it over the top almost to the edge
12. Decorate using fruits of your choice

Tuscan Grape Cake

Preparation time: 10 minutes
Cooking time: 45 minutes
Serves 12

Ingredients:

- ¾ cup all-purpose flour
- ½ cup ground almond
- ½ cup corn meal
- 2 tsp baking powder
- ½ tsp salt
- 1/3 cup vegetable oil
- ¾ cup brown sugar, light variety
- 1 tsp almond extract
- 3 eggs
- ½ cup sour cream
- 2 cups seedless red grapes
- 1 tbsp. brown sugar
- 1 tbsp. white sugar

Instructions:

1. Preheat the oven to 350° F
2. Blend the almonds, flour, salt, baking powder and cornmeal together
3. In another bowl, mix together the light brown sugar, almond extract, and the oil
4. Add in the eggs, beating them in one at a time
5. Add the cream, whisking to combine
6. Add the flour mixture in and combine well
7. Grease a 9-inch springform pan and pour the mixture in evenly
8. Bake for 10 minutes

9. Remove the cake from the oven and spread the grapes in an even layer over the top
10. Mix together the brown and white sugars, sprinkle over the top and bake for a further 30 to 35 minutes
11. Leave to cool completely before cutting to serve

Chapter 11: Snacks

Marinated Olives with Feta Cheese

Preparation time: 70 minutes
Serves 12
Ingredients:

- 1 cup of olives, pitted and sliced
- ½ cup feta cheese, diced
- 2 tbsp. extra virgin olive oil
- Juice and zest of one lemon
- 2 sliced garlic cloves
- 1 tsp fresh chopped rosemary
- Fresh ground black pepper for seasoning
- Pinch of crushed red pepper

Instructions:
1. Combine all of the ingredients together in a bowl
2. Cover the bowl and refrigerate for 24 hours before serving

Hummus

Preparation time: 5 minutes
Serves 4

Ingredients:

- 1 16 oz. can rinsed and drained chickpeas
- 1/3 cup fat-free plain yogurt
- ¼ cup scallions, minced
- ¼ cup finely minced fresh parsley
- Juice from 2 lemons
- 5 tsp tahini
- 1 tbsp. olive oil
- 3 minced garlic cloves
- 1/8 tsp ground black pepper
- Low salt soy sauce
- Ground red pepper

Instructions:

1. Put the chickpeas in a blender and blend until smooth
2. Scrape the sides occasionally to make sure it is all combined
3. Add the scallions, yogurt, parsley, tahini, juice, garlic, oil, black pepper, and a splash of soy sauce
4. Process until you have a smooth creamy consistency – add a little water if needed
5. Spoon into a serving bowl, sprinkle red pepper and serve with crudités for dipping

Cherries with Ricotta & Toasted Almonds

Preparation time: 5 minutes
Cooking time: 1-2 minutes
Serves 1

Ingredients:
- ¾ cup pitted cherries, frozen
- 2 tbsp. ricotta, part-skim
- 1 tbsp. slivered toasted almonds

Instructions:
1. Warm the cherries in a bowl in the microwave for a couple of minutes
2. Layer the cherries in a bowl and top off with the ricotta and almonds

Tomato & Basil Finger Sandwiches

Preparation time: 5 minutes
Serves 4

Ingredients:
- 4 slices bread, whole grain
- 8 tsp mayonnaise, low-fat
- 4 thick tomato slices
- 4 tsp fresh sliced basil
- 1/8 tsp salt
- 1/8 tsp. ground black pepper

Instructions:
1. Cut rounds from the bread that are a little larger than your tomato slices
2. Spread mayonnaise over each slice
3. Layer the tomato and basil on top and season with salt and pepper

Date Wraps

Preparation time: 10 minutes
Serves 4

Ingredients:
- 16 whole dates, pitted
- 16 prosciutto slices
- Ground pepper for seasoning

Instructions:
1. Wrap each date in a slice of prosciutto
2. Season with pepper

Blueberries with Lemon Cream

Preparation time: 10 minutes
Serves 4

Ingredients:
- 4 oz. cream cheese, low fat
- ¾ cup vanilla yogurt, low fat
- 1 tsp honey
- 2 tsp lemon zest
- 2 cups fresh blueberries

Instructions:
1. Break the cream cheese up in a bowl, using a fork
2. Drain the yogurt to discard any excess liquid and add the yogurt and the honey to the cream cheese
3. Beat with an electric mixer until creamy and light
4. Stir the lemon zest in
5. Layer the cream and the blueberries in dessert dishes and, if not eating straight away, cover and cool in the refrigerator for about 8 hour

Conclusion

Thank you again for purchasing this book!

I hope this book was able to help you to understand the underlying principles of the Mediterranean diet and how it can help you to lose weight and keep it off for good. The Mediterranean diet is a healthy one and is full of fresh, whole foods and wonderful, easy to prepare recipes that you can enjoy with abandon, without having to worry about becoming obsessed with counting calories. The very nature of the diet means that you will find it easier to lose the excess pounds and feel great while you are doing it. Not all of the recipes are straightforward but most of them are simple to prepare and cook and the effort will most definitely be worthwhile.

The next step is to, quite simply, start the diet! Make your shopping list from the list of foods provided for you and head off to the store. Like any diet, you may find it difficult to change your eating habits but, once you get into it, you will find it easy to stick to and follow. Change your life today; lose weight, and improve your health and energy levels no end by taking up the challenge of the Mediterranean diet a new lifestyle, a new you.

KETOGENIC DIET

Step By Step Guide And 70

+

Low Carb, Proven Recipes For Rapid Weight Loss

Table of Contents

Introduction

All of us have too much to do and too little time. In the process of getting everything done, we often lose focus on the more important aspects of our life. One of these is probably the one thing that you should pay the most attention to, namely, health.

Being healthy is crucial to living a happy and fulfilling life. If your body is not treated right, you will soon have to face the ramifications. Just by making a few better choices in your daily life, you will see the difference it makes to everything. Just because you're always in a rush does not mean you have to skip meals or eat just anything that you can get your hands on.

Food is important for your body and the right kind of food will do you a world of good. You do not have to make any drastic changes in your diet or starve yourself either. There are a lot of fad diets and methods that claim to help you lose weight fast or get healthier than ever. Learn more about what is good for your body and what is actually going to harm you. We'll help you out with one such diet that actually works and will help you work steadily towards a healthier body.

Here you will learn all about the ketogenic diet. You might already have heard of it but may not know what it entails. We will tell you all you need to know about what it is and how it helps you. Stop following random fads that do not work or that harm your body.

As you read on, you will understand exactly why a lot of people vouch for this particular diet. You will soon be a follower as well.

Chapter 1: What Is The Ketogenic Diet?

The ketogenic or keto diet has gained quite a bit of popularity over that past few years. It is basically a diet that is quite low in carbohydrate and high in fats. The diet will help you lower blood sugar as well as insulin levels in the body. Your body's metabolism will focus on fats instead of carbohydrates for providing the energy it needs.

The ketones produced in your liver will be used for providing energy to your body. The carbohydrate intake is reduced drastically and replaced with fat. This forces your body to go into a state of ketosis. In turn, your body becomes much more efficient at burning fat and using it for energy instead of depending on carbohydrates. The fat in the liver is also converted to ketones which supply the brain with energy.

We will explain how it works further. Eating a high carbohydrate diet will make your body produce more of glucose and insulin. Since glucose is the easiest molecule to break down, the body chooses to use it as a source of energy instead of any fat that you eat. This forces the fat to get stored and makes you gain weight. However, now that you reduce the intake of carbohydrates, your body is forced to undergo ketosis. It is a natural mechanism of the body wherein the fats in the liver are broken down to produce ketones. This metabolic state is what helps you use the stored fat in your body as the main source of energy now.

There are different variants of the keto diet that you can follow:

> The standard ketogenic diet has very low carbohydrates, moderate protein content and high amount of fat.

➤ The high protein ketogenic diet has a higher amount of proteins than the standard diet.

➤ The targeted ketogenic diet involves adding carbohydrates in your diet according to your workout schedule.

➤ The cyclical ketogenic diet has a cycle where you follow the ketogenic diet for a certain number of days and then add carbs for a couple of days before switching back.

Let's take a look at how you can follow this diet. We have put together a list of food you should eat and those that should be avoided. This will help you keep track of what you eat and how to stay on the diet correctly.

You need to avoid most food which is carbohydrate based. List of food to avoid:

- Potatoes, carrots and other tubers or root vegetables.

- Processed vegetable oils

- Alcohol

- Diet or low-fat products

- Fruits

- Grains and starches like rice, pasta, cereal, etc.

- Lentils, peas, chickpeas and other beans or legumes

- Sugar-free foods

Eat food that is low carb but has enough proteins and fats. List of food to eat:

- Low carb vegetables like tomatoes and onions

- Nuts and seeds like chia seeds, almonds, flaxseeds, etc.

- Eggs

- Chicken, bacon, turkey, red meat, ham

- Grass-fed butter and cream

- Healthy oils like olive oil, coconut oil, avocado oil

- Avocados or guacamole

- Unprocessed cheese

- Salmon, trout, mackerel and other fatty fish

- Leafy greens like kale and spinach

The list of what to eat and what to avoid will help you choose your food. Stay away from anything which isn't keto friendly and you will soon see results. There are so many recipes which help you stay on this diet without it getting monotonous. You can try different keto recipes to help you prepare the right meals for your diet and to eat something delicious and new every day. When you get hungry in between meals, eat a small portion of some keto friendly food. For instance, you can eat dark chocolate, strawberries, salsa and guacamole, boiled eggs, nuts, cheese or some yogurt.

The diet does not require you to starve yourself or give up all the food that you like. You just need to cut out a few things that you might normally eat and eat some other foods instead. If you are worried about eating out, we can help you as well. If you order a burger, don't eat the bun. Choose a meat or fish main course. Dessert can be some berries and cream or cheeses. Egg-based dishes are also a good choice. It isn't actually that hard once you stick to the basics whether it is at home or while eating at a restaurant. The changes you make on this diet are easy to maintain and show you results soon enough.

Once you start the diet, just be aware of a few things to avoid any problems.

Precautions:

➤ Keto flu is seen to occur in some people when they start the diet. The symptoms include low energy levels, sleeping problems, nausea and increased hunger pangs. It passes after a couple of weeks. You can start by reducing the carbs little by little instead of totally cutting them out of your diet.

➤ The water and mineral content in your body is affected as well so add more salt and supplements to your diet to help balance this.

➤ Eat your meals until you are full and do not try to eat less while on this diet just to lose weight faster.

➤ Certain supplements like whey, caffeine and creatine can help you ease into the diet.

The ketogenic diet is a great option for most people and is shown to be highly effective. However, if you are suffering from certain diseases or ailments, it is advised that you consult your doctor first. Making dietary changes can affect your treatment and body as well. If they say it is okay, then go ahead with it. The diet is effective if you follow it properly and consistently for some time. It won't show results in a day or two but will have long lasting effects that you will benefit from.

Chapter 2: How Does The Diet Help You Stay Healthy And Why One Should Follow It?

A number of reasons can be stated to convince anyone to follow the ketogenic diet. Just about any issue like weight loss to medical treatments is dealt with using this particular diet. Thus you can say that it is a diet for everyone. We have put together a list of all the benefits you will reap by following the keto diet.

> Weight loss is one of the main reasons why people go on this diet. Since the body uses fat for energy, it helps in losing a lot of the weight from your body. Your insulin levels drop on this diet and this prompts more fat to be burnt and this helps you lose weight. It has been found to be even more effective than a diet where you reduce the fat consumption a lot.

> Diabetes is an ailment that affects a lot of people and this diet helps them as well. Excess fat in the body is linked to prediabetes as well as type-2 diabetes. Your insulin sensitivity increases a lot when you go on the ketogenic diet and this helps to deal with these conditions. You also lose a lot of weight and all this helps in treating diabetic conditions on a huge scale.

> Energy levels increase and you become much more productive in return. Fats are a more satisfying source of food to consume and a very effective source of energy as well. This helps in keeping you sated and energetic at the same time all day long.

> Brain function or focus is improved a lot. Ketones

produced while on this diet will provide fuel for the brain. The blood sugar levels in your body are also balanced better. This helps in improving the concentration levels of a person on the keto diet.

➢ Epilepsy is one of the main advocates of the ketogenic diet. Children afflicted with epilepsy are treated by using this diet as a form of therapy. It has been found to be effective and has been used for a very long time now. With the help of the keto diet, patients can reduce the amount of medication they require and feel much better overall.

➢ Acne is a common problem for most people at some age or the other. The keto diet helps in lowering insulin levels and involves less sugar consumption. This is why it helps deal with acne as well.

➢ Cholesterol and Blood Pressure needs to be maintained in any person. The keto diet helps in increasing HDL and decreasing LDL. The loss in weight also helps to lower high blood pressure.

➢ Insulin resistance can cause a lot of issues. The keto diet helps in increasing insulin sensitivity and thus deals with this condition. This can help prevent diabetes.

➢ Heart diseases are linked to blood pressure, body fat and blood sugar levels. The keto diet aids in maintaining the right levels in the body and thus prevents heart diseases from occurring.

As you can see, there are a number of benefits to gain by following the simple ketogenic diet. These results are why a lot of people swear by this diet and you should try it out as well.

Chapter 3: Breakfast Recipes

Spinach Mushroom & Feta Crust less Quiche

Serves: 3

Ingredients

- 4 oz. button mushrooms, sliced
- 5 oz. frozen spinach, thawed
- 1 clove garlic, minced
- ½ cup milk
- 2 large eggs, whisked
- 2 tablespoons parmesan, grated
- 1 oz. feta cheese
- ¼ cup mozzarella grated
- Salt & pepper to taste

Method:

1. Preheat the oven to 350 F. Press & remove the excess moisture from the spinach.
2. Place a non-stick skillet on medium heat and spray cooking spray over it. Add mushroom and garlic and sauté until gets fully cooked and become soft.
3. Grease a pie dish with cooking spray. Spread the spinach on the pie dish and layer it with sautéed mushrooms. Top it up with crumbled feta cheese.
4. Mix together Parmesan, milk and whisked eggs. Add pepper and stir.
5. Pour into the pie dish. Sprinkle mozzarella over it.
6. Place a baking sheet in the oven and put the pie dish over it and bake until golden brown.
7. Slice and serve.

Spinach Cucumber Smoothie

Ingredients:

- 2 cups spinach
- 1 cucumber (cubed)
- 1 cup coconut milk, unsweetened
- 15 drops liquid Stevia
- ½ teaspoon xanthan gum
- 2 tablespoons of MCT oil
- 8 ice cubes

Method:

1. Wash and shred the spinach leaves.
2. In the blender, add the shredded spinach leaves and cubed cucumber.
3. Pour the unsweetened coconut milk and liquid Stevia into the blender.
4. To this mixture add half teaspoon of xanthan gum and 2 tablespoons of MCT oil.
5. Add ice cubes to the blender and mix gently using a ladle.
6. Blend for 2 minutes. The spinach shreds give this drink a wonderful texture.
7. Serve immediately.

Tomato Broccoli Frittata

Serves: 3

Ingredients

- 5 eggs, whisked
- 1 tablespoon olive oil
- 1 ounce gouda cheese, crumbled
- 1 small head broccoli, chopped into small florets
- 1 medium tomato, chopped
- 1/2 teaspoon pepper powder
- 1 small avocado, peeled, pitted, sliced

Method:

1. Add eggs, broccoli, tomato, salt and pepper to a bowl and whisk well.
2. Add cheese and mix until well combined.
3. Place an ovenproof pan over medium heat. Add oil and swirl the pan so that the oil spreads.
4. Add the egg mixture and cook until the sides are slightly set.
5. Remove from heat.
6. Bake in a preheated oven at 425 degrees F for about 20-30 minutes or until golden brown.
7. Slice and serve with avocado slices.

French toast

Serves: 9

Ingredients:

<u>For protein bread:</u>

- 6 eggs separated
- 2 oz. cream cheese
- ½ cup egg white

<u>For French toast:</u>

- 1 egg
- ½ teaspoon vanilla
- ¼ cup coconut milk or almond milk
- ½ teaspoon cinnamon powder.

<u>For syrup:</u>

- ¼ cup butter
- ¼ cup almond milk
- ¼ cup swerve confectioners.

Method:

1. To make bread: Beat the egg whites until very stiff.
2. Add protein powder into the egg whites and mix gently. Add cream cheese and fold gently.
3. Grease a bread pan and pour the dough into it.
4. Put it in the preheated oven at 325 degrees F and bake it until golden brown.
5. Slice the bread when completely cooled down. Make 9 slices.
6. To make French toast: Put a greased skillet on medium high flame.
7. Mix 1 egg, almond milk, vanilla and cinnamon in a bowl.

8. Coat bread slices with egg whites.
9. Grill bread slices on hot skillets until golden brown. Repeat with remaining slices.
10. To make syrup: Melt butter over high heat in a saucepan. Add swerve and milk immediately. Whisk constantly until smooth. Remove from heat and cool. Store in an airtight container in the refrigerator.
11. Top French toast with syrup and serve.

Mini Santé Fe Frittata's

Serves: 4

Ingredients:

- 5 large eggs
- 1 egg white
- 4 ounces pork sausage
- 1/4 cup milk
- 1/2 cup red bell pepper, coarsely chopped in small cubes
- 1/2 cup yellow bell pepper, coarsely chopped in small cubes
- 1/4 cup pepper Jack cheese
- Salt to taste
- Pepper powder to taste
- 1 onion, sliced
- 2 tablespoons fresh cilantro, chopped

Method:

1. Place a skillet over medium heat. Add the sausages and cook until done.
2. Remove with a slotted spoon and set aside. Crumble it when it is cooled.
3. Place the skillet back on heat. Add peppers and cook until tender. Remove from heat and set aside.
4. Add eggs, egg white and milk to a bowl and whisk well.
5. Take 6 muffin cups and grease it with a little butter or oil. Add bacon to the cups. Next layer with bell peppers.
6. Next layer with the egg mixture and finally top with cheese. Stir lightly with a fork.
7. Bake in a preheated oven at 350 degrees F for about 20-30 minutes or until it browns. Remove from the oven.
8. Loosen the edges with a knife. Invert on to a plate and serve.

Kiwi Avocado Smoothie

Ingredients:

- 2 avocados
- 1/2 cup coconut milk.
- 1/2 cup kiwis
- 1 scoop whey powder, vanilla flavored
- 1 tablespoon chia seeds
- 6 drops liquid Stevia
- 1/2 cup water
- 3 ice cubes
- Cinnamon Powder (for garnish, optional)

Method:

1. Scoop the avocados and keep aside.
2. Add the avocados and half a cup of coconut milk to a blender.
3. Add half a cup of freshly cut kiwis to the mixture and 1 scoop of vanilla flavored whey protein powder. Blend for 30 seconds on medium.
4. Add the chia seeds and liquid Stevia to the mixture in the blender.
5. Pour half a cup of water and ice cubes into the blender.
6. Blend at medium speed until smooth.
7. Garnish with cinnamon powder and serve chilled.

Middle Eastern Shakshuka

Serves: 6

Ingredients:

- 18 ounces stew meat
- 5 cloves garlic, sliced
- 1 large onion, chopped
- 3 poblano peppers, chopped
- 1 large red bell pepper, chopped
- 1 large green bell pepper, chopped
- 2 bay leaves
- 1 ½ teaspoons paprika
- 1 ½ teaspoons ground cumin
- ¾ teaspoon crushed red pepper flakes
- Salt to taste
- Pepper to taste
- 3 tablespoons extra virgin olive oil
- ¾ cup tomato sauce
- 1 ½ cans (15 ounces each) diced tomatoes

Method:

1. Mix together in a large bowl, cumin, paprika, salt and pepper. Add meat and toss until well coated.
2. Heat and pan on medium flame and add oil. When the oil is heated, add beef with the spices and sauté until light brown.
3. Add onions, bell pepper, poblano pepper and garlic and sauté until onions are translucent.
4. Add bay leaves, crushed red pepper, and tomatoes with its juice and mash lightly the tomatoes. Stir well and cook on medium heat for 20 minutes.
5. Once the beef is cooked, discard the bay leaf and tomato sauce. Stir well. Taste and adjust the seasoning if necessary.

6. Make 6 cavities in the mixture. Crack an egg into each. Cover and cook for the remaining cook time or until the eggs are cooked as per your desire.

Italian Omelet

Ingredients

- 6 eggs
- 3 ounces full fat Brie cheese, sliced
- 3 tablespoons butter
- 15 Kalamata olives, pitted
- 3 tablespoons MCT oil
- 1/2 teaspoon salt
- 1 1/2 teaspoons Herbes De Provence
- 1 large avocado, peeled, pitted, cut into thick slices

Method

1. Add eggs, oil, herbes de Provence, olives and salt. Whisk well.
2. Place a nonstick skillet over medium - high heat. Add butter. When the butter melts, add avocado and fry until golden brown all over. Remove and set aside.
3. Place the skillet back on high heat. Add the egg mixture into it.
4. Place the cheese slice on the egg. Cover and cook until the underside is golden brown.
5. Flip sides and cook the other side too. Remove from the pan.
6. Slice into 6 wedges. Top with avocado slices and serve.

Keto Kale Herbs Smoothie

Ingredients

- 1 bunch kale
- 1 teaspoon salt
- 2 tablespoons collagen
- 2 teaspoons of apple cider vinegar
- 1 teaspoons of oregano powder
- 2 teaspoons butter
- 10 drops of MCT oil

Directions:

1. Take a bunch of kale and wash it clean under running water.
2. Cook in a steam cooker for about 8 minutes. Allow the kale to cool for a while.
3. Drain the water and add it to the blender.
4. Add a teaspoon of salt and a couple of tablespoons of collagen.
5. Take two tablespoons of apple cider vinegar and add it to the mixture and mix it well.
6. Now add a seasoning of a teaspoon of oregano powder. Along with the seasoning add 3 teaspoons of butter and 10 drops of MCT oil.
7. Switch on the blender and blend the ingredients for two minutes until the mixture is smooth in texture.
8. Serve immediately

Flax Sandwich Buns

Serves: 3

Ingredients

- 9 tablespoons flaxseed meal
- 1 teaspoon caraway seeds
- 2 teaspoons onion powder
- 3 large eggs
- 1 teaspoon baking powder
- 1 1/2 tablespoons water
- 2 drops Stevia
- 1 1/2 tablespoons olive oil

Method

1. Mix together all the dry ingredients in a bowl.
2. Mix together all the wet ingredients in a bowl.
3. Pour the wet ingredients into the bowl of dry ingredients and mix well.
4. Pour into greased muffin pan (Fill up to 2/3)
5. Bake in a preheated oven at 325 degrees F for about 15 minutes or until it done.
6. Slit in the middle, horizontally. Serve with toppings of your choice.

Vanilla Pumpkin Squash Smoothie

Ingredients:

- 1 medium pumpkin
- 1/2 cup whey powder, vanilla flavored
- 1 teaspoon vanilla essence
- 2 cups almond milk

Method:

1. Preheat oven to 300 degrees Fahrenheit.
2. Halve the pumpkins and keep both the halves face down in a baking tray.
3. Bake until tender (about half an hour.) Remove the pumpkin halves from the oven and insert a needle or fork to check if done.
4. Allow to cool for a few minutes.
5. Once cooled, remove seeds using a spoon.
6. Scoop out the pumpkin flesh into a big bowl.
7. Add whey powder and vanilla essence to this mixture.
8. Blend for 2 minutes at medium speed until smooth and then add in the almond milk and blend for another minute.
9. Pour into glasses and refrigerate. This smoothie can be stored for up to a week.

Eggs Baked In a Skillet

Serves: 2

Ingredients:

- 1/3 cup plain Greek yogurt
- 1 tablespoon unsalted butter, divided
- 2 tablespoons leek, chopped
- 1 clove garlic, halved
- Salt to taste
- 1 tablespoon olive oil
- 1 scallion, chopped
- 1 teaspoon fresh lemon juice
- 5 cups fresh spinach, chopped
- ½ teaspoon fresh oregano, chopped
- Crushed red pepper flakes to taste
- 2 large eggs

Method:

1. Add garlic & salt to the bowl of yogurt and set aside for some time.
2. Place a heavy skillet on medium heat. Add half the butter, when butter melts add leek and scallion.
3. Lower the heat. Sauté until it becomes tender.
4. Increase heat. Add spinach, lemon juice & salt. Sauté until spinach wilts.
5. Transfer the mixture into an ovenproof skillet. Make 2 deep cavities in the skillet.
6. Break eggs carefully in each cavity. Sprinkle salt over it. Place the skillet in a preheated oven at 300 degrees F and bake until the eggs set.
7. Place a small saucepan with remaining butter over medium low heat. Add red pepper flakes and salt. When it becomes frothy, add oregano and cook for 30 seconds and remove from heat.

8. Remove garlic from yogurt. Top the spinach & eggs with yogurt and sprinkle spiced butter over it.
9. Serve.

Taiwanese Oyster Omelet

Serves: 1

Ingredients:

- 2 ounces shelled oyster with juice
- ½ teaspoon arrowroot powder
- 1 tablespoon sweet potato starch
- 1 egg
- 2 teaspoons lard
- 2 teaspoons olive oil
- 1/8 teaspoon sesame oil
- 2 teaspoons peanut oil
- 1 tablespoon green onion, minced
- 1/3 cup baby bok Choy leaves, separated
- White pepper powder to taste
- Salt to taste

For the omelet sauce:
- ½ teaspoon ketchup
- ½ teaspoon hoisin sauce
- 1/8 teaspoon rice vinegar
- ¼ teaspoon Sriracha sauce
- ¼ teaspoon Chinese fine chili sauce

Method:

1. To make omelet sauce: Add all the ingredients of the omelet sauce into a bowl along with a teaspoon of boiling water. Stir and set aside.
2. Retain about 2 teaspoons of the liquid and drain the oysters.
3. Add sweet potato starch, arrowroot powder, salt, oyster

liquid, and 1-teaspoon water into a bowl and mix well.

4. Add eggs, salt, pepper and sesame oil into another bowl and whisk well.
5. Heat a pan on medium flame. Add lard. When lard melts, add bok Choy and sauté until it wilts.
6. Pour the sauce mixture over it. Sprinkle oysters over it. Let it cook until the mixture turns transparent.
7. Pour egg mixture over it.
8. Close the lid. Cook for 2 mins under steam and then uncover and remove on a plate.
9. Garnish with green onions and serve.

Broccoli and Cheese Omelet

Serves - 2

Ingredients:

- 4 egg whites
- 2 eggs
- 1 cup broccoli, chopped into small pieces, cooked
- 2 tablespoons almond milk
- Salt to taste
- Pepper powder to taste
- 2 slices Swiss cheese
- Cooking spray

Method:

1. Add eggs, whites, milk, salt and pepper to a bowl and whisk well.
2. Place a nonstick skillet over medium heat. Spray with cooking spray.
3. When the pan is heated, add half the egg mixture. Swirl the pan so that the egg spreads.
4. Place a slice of cheese at the center of the omelet. Place half the broccoli over the cheese.
5. Cook until the egg sets. Fold the sides over the broccoli. Remove on to a plate and serve.
6. Repeat the above 3 steps with the remaining eggs and broccoli.

Chocolate Sesame Smoothie

Ingredients

- 2 scoops of low carbohydrate powdered protein
- 2 teaspoons cocoa powder, unsweetened
- 1 teaspoon husk from psyllium
- 300 ml water
- 2 tablespoons sesame oil
- 5 drops liquid sweetening agent
- 200 ml cooking cream, with no more than 35g of fat

Method:

1. Mix the protein powder, cocoa powder, and psyllium husk in a large glass.
2. To this mixture, add about 300ml water and shake well until it is smooth. (You can alternatively use a blender for the same, but works well in a glass too)
3. To this, add 2 tablespoons of sesame oil and the liquid sweetening agent. (The sesame oil provides valuable nutrients to the shake while giving it a nutty texture.)
4. Scoop the cooking cream and add it to the mixture. Do not shake but gently mix until the ingredients are homogenous.
5. Add ice cubes and consume within half an hour.

Cinnamon Muffins

Serves - 4

Ingredients

For the muffins:
- 1/2 cup coconut flour
- 6 eggs
- 4 tablespoons flaxseed powder
- 20 walnuts, chopped
- 1 cup plain yogurt
- 4 tablespoons almond milk
- 1/2 cup sugar free maple syrup
- 1/2 teaspoon soda
- 1/2 teaspoon salt
- 4 teaspoons ground cinnamon

For the glaze:
- 4 tablespoons butter, melted
- 1/2 cup sugar free maple syrup
- 4 teaspoons ground cinnamon

Method

1. To make muffins: Mix together all the dry ingredients in a bowl.
2. Mix together all the wet ingredients in a bowl.
3. Add the dry ingredients to the wet ingredients and whisk well.
4. Pour into greased muffin cups (fill up to 3/4).
5. Bake in a preheated oven at 350 degrees F for about 20-30 minutes or until it turns light brown. Remove from the oven and set aside to cool for about 10 minutes.
6. Meanwhile, mix together the ingredients of the glaze.
7. Loosen the edges with a knife. Invert on to a plate and brush with the glaze.
8. Serve warm.

Chapter 4: Soup & Salad Recipes
Spicy Thai Shrimp Salad

Serves: 6

Ingredients:

- 1 ½ pounds small shrimp, peeled, deveined
- 6 teaspoons fish sauce
- 3 tablespoons lime juice
- 1 ½ tablespoons olive oil
- Stevia drops to taste
- 1 medium red bell pepper, thinly sliced
- 1 medium yellow bell pepper, thinly sliced
- 2 medium cucumbers, thinly sliced
- Salt to taste
- ½ teaspoon red crushed pepper
- 2 tablespoons fresh basil, minced
- 2 tablespoons fresh mint, minced
- 2 tablespoons fresh cilantro, minced

Method:

1. Sauté the shrimp on medium heat for about 2 mins until they get cooked.
2. You can even just steam them if you prefer it that way.
3. Transfer the shrimp to a bowl. Add rest of the ingredients and mix well.
4. Serve!

Chicken Salad Stuffed Avocado

Serves 2:

Ingredients:

- 6 oz. chicken breast
- 2 tablespoon diced onions
- 2 avocadoes
- 2 stalk celery
- 2/3 cup sour cream
- Salt and pepper as per taste

Method:

1. On low heat cook the chicken breast until it gets tender. Shred the chicken with help of forks.
2. In a bowl mix chicken, red onion and celery.
3. Cut & scoop out some avocado and add in the chicken mixture.
4. Mix the sour cream and add salt & pepper.
5. Fill the avocado halves with the mixture and serve.

Strawberry Zoodle Salad with Goat cheese and Pistachios

Serves 2

Ingredients:

<u>For the salad:</u>

- 2 strawberries, sliced
- 2 cups zucchini noodles
- 2 tablespoons herbed goat cheese, sliced and crumbled
- 2 tablespoons pistachios

<u>For dressing:</u>

- 8 strawberries
- 4 tablespoons avocado oil
- 4 tablespoons balsamic vinegar
- 1 teaspoon garlic, minced
- ¼ teaspoon salt
- ¼ teaspoon freshly cracked pepper

Method:

1. Mix salad ingredients in a bowl.
2. Place dressing ingredients in a blender and blend until well combined.
3. Toss the salad with 2 tablespoon of strawberry balsamic dressing and serve.

Salmon Salad

Serves: 4

Ingredients:

- 3 stalks celery, thinly sliced
- 2 shallots, minced
- 2 cloves of garlic, minced
- 1 bell pepper, thinly sliced
- 1 medium cucumber
- ½ pint tomatoes
- ¼ olive oil or to taste
- Juice of ½ a lemon
- Zest of ½ a lemon
- 1 tablespoon red wine vinegar
- ½ teaspoon kosher salt or to taste
- ½ teaspoon fresh or dried dill
- ¼ teaspoon freshly ground black pepper
- ¼ teaspoon smoked paprika
- ¼ teaspoon ground cumin
- ¼ teaspoon crushed red pepper flakes
- 2 cans salmon, drained

Method:

1. Halve the cucumber lengthwise and then slice it. Halve the tomatoes.
2. Add all the ingredients to a large bowl. Toss well and refrigerate for an hour.
3. Add more seasoning if necessary and serve.

Spinach and Bacon Salad

Serves: 3

Ingredients:

- 4 cups raw spinach
- ½ cup chopped shallots
- 6 slices bacon
- 1 tbsp. butter

Method:

1. First slice the bacon strips finely. Melt butter on a skillet placed on medium flame.
2. Add the shallots and the bacon to the skillet. Sauté until the shallots have turned golden brown and are translucent.
3. Now, add the spinach and cook until the leaves have wilted. Toss the ingredients and serve hot.

Thai Style Chicken Salad

Serves: 3

Ingredients:

- 1 shallot, minced
- 3 tablespoons mayonnaise
- 3 tablespoons nonfat plain yogurt
- 1 teaspoon lemon juice
- 1 tablespoon chili sauce
- 3 cups chicken, skinless, boneless, chopped
- 1 teaspoon lemon juice
- Pepper powder to taste
- Salt to taste
- 1 small red bell pepper, chopped
- ½ cup Napa cabbage, thinly sliced
- 2 tablespoons cashews, chopped, toasted
- 1-tablespoon peanut oil.

Method:

1. Stir-fry the chicken on medium heat using some peanut oil.
2. Mix the rest of the ingredients and toss the stir-fried chicken in it.
3. Serve.

Chicken, Tomato and Bacon Salad

Ingredients

For the Salad

- 2 large uncooked chicken breasts (cut them into chunks that are one inch each)
- 4 tsp. Canadian Steak Brand (you could use any brand that you want)
- 4 tbsp. butter
- 10 slices bacon
- 2 small tomatoes
- 3 ounces Muenster cheese

For the dressing

- 3 tbsp. butter
- 2 raw eggs (preferably eggs from a pastured chicken. This egg will be richer)
- 3 ounces mayonnaise
- 3 tsp. lemon juice
- 1 tsp. salt

Method

The Salad

1. Add the Canadian steak seasoning to the chicken and spread it neatly.
2. Take a pan and place it on a medium flame and add the butter. When the butter begins to melt, add the chicken breasts and sauté it.
3. Make sure that it is cooked through before you remove it off the pan. Leave it aside to cool down to room

temperature.

4. Cut the bacon into thin strips. Sauté the strips in a pan on a medium flame until you drain all the oil.

The Dressing

1. Take a small pan and add the butter to it. Place the pan on low heat. Once the butter melts pull the pan off the flame and leave the butter to cool.
2. Add the yolk to the butter and whisk the two well until the mixture has become glossy and smooth.
3. Add the remaining ingredients and whisk until the mixture is smooth.

The finished Salad

1. Take a plate and add all the ingredients and the dressing and mix them well.
2. Ensure that the ingredients are coated well with the dressing.

Coconut Lime Chicken & Snow Peas Salad

Serves: 4

Ingredients:

- 16 ounces chicken tenders
- 2 cups light coconut milk
- Stevia drops to taste
- ½ cup lime juice
- 8 romaine lettuce, shredded
- 2 cups snow peas, sliced
- 2 cups red cabbage, shredded
- ¼ cup red onion, minced
- 1/3 cup fresh cilantro, chopped
- 1 teaspoon salt or to taste

Method:

1. Whisk together in a large bowl, coconut milk, Stevia, lime juice, and salt. Pour ¾ of it into a bowl.
2. Add chicken and stir.
3. Let it sit for 30 mins and then transfer the mix to a pan. Cook the chicken in the same juice on a medium flame. Allow it to soak in most of the juices as it cooks.
4. Remove the chicken with a slotted spoon. When cool enough to handle, slice the chicken.
5. Add vegetables into the large dish, which has ¼ the dressing. Toss well.
6. Divide and place the salad on individual serving plates. Place the chicken slices over it. Ladle a little of the cooked liquid over it and serve.

Lobster Salad

Serves: 4

Ingredients:

- 1 1/2 pounds Northern lobster (steamed)
- 4 cup Chinese cabbage (Bok-Choy or Pak-Choi), shredded
- 1 small red peppers
- 8 medium spring onions
- 2 tablespoons sesame seeds
- Salt to taste
- Pepper powder to taste

For the dressing:
- 4 tablespoons rice vinegar
- 4 tablespoons tamari sauce
- 2 tablespoons canola oil
- 2 teaspoons sesame oil
- 2 teaspoons ginger, minced

Method:

1. To make the dressing: Mix together all the ingredients of the dressing in jar and shake vigorously.
2. Mix together rest of the ingredients in a large bowl. Pour dressing over the salad. Toss well and serve.

Cream of Broccoli Soup

Serves 3

Ingredients:

- 1 red onion, chopped chunky
- ½ teaspoon tamari sauce
- 1 tablespoon coconut oil
- 2.5 cup of water
- 1 cup of fresh Broccoli florets
- ½ tablespoon Chicken soup powder
- ½ cup of whipping cream.

Method:

1. Heat coconut oil in a pan and sauté red onions in it.
2. Add broccoli and water. Cook for 10 minutes.
3. Put the soup in a blender and make puree.
4. Lower the heat and add cream. Stir
5. Serve hot in soup bowls.

Thai Hot and Sour Shrimp Soup

Serves: 2

Ingredients:

- 8 to 10 shrimp, peeled, with its tail on, and deveined, set aside the shells
- 1 small onion, chopped
- 1 tablespoon coconut oil, divided
- 1 inch piece galangal, peeled, chopped into thick slices
- 2 cloves garlic
- 2 fresh kaffir leaves or ¼ teaspoon lemon zest, grated
- 1 stalk lemon grass, chopped into 1 inch pieces
- 1 Thai red chili, roughly chopped
- ¼ pound crimini or shiitake or oyster or button mushrooms, rinsed, sliced into wedges
- 2 ½ cups chicken broth
- 1 tablespoon fresh lime juice
- ½ small green zucchini, sliced
- Salt to taste
- Pepper to taste
- 1 tablespoon fish sauce
- 1 tablespoon fresh lime juice
- 2 tablespoons fresh basil, chopped
- 2 tablespoons fresh cilantro, chopped
- Salt to taste
- Pepper to taste

Method:

1. Heat a pan on medium flame. Add ½ tablespoon coconut oil. When the oil is heated, add shrimp shells that were kept aside and stir constantly until they turn red in color.
2. Add onions, galangal, garlic, lemon grass, kaffir lime

leaves or fresh lime zest, Thai red chili, salt and pepper. Sauté for a few minutes until the onions turn translucent.

3. Add broth and stir.
4. Let the mix cook for 10 mins or until everything gets well incorporated and cooked.
5. Remove the shrimp shells with a slotted spoon. Discard the shells.
6. Transfer the stock into a bowl and set aside.
7. Add the remaining coconut oil into a pot.
8. When the oil is heated, add zucchini slices and mushroom and season with salt and pepper. Sauté for a few minutes until tender.
9. Add the cooked broth into the pot. Add shrimp into the pot and stir. Let it cook for another 5 – 7 minutes.
10. Add lime juice, salt, pepper, and fish sauce. Stir well. Taste and adjust the seasoning if necessary.
11. Simmer for a couple of minutes or until the shrimp is cooked. Add fresh cilantro and basil and stir.
12. Ladle into soup bowls and serve immediately.

Mallow Soup

Serves: 3

Ingredients:

- 3 cups water
- 3 pieces chicken, bite sized
- 1 chicken bouillon cube
- 1 small onion, chopped
- 1 package (14 ounces) frozen Moulkhia, minced or chopped
- ½ teaspoon ground allspice
- 2 cloves garlic
- 2 tablespoons olive oil

Method:

1. Heat the oil in a pan and sauté the onions in it. When the onions turn translucent, ass the chicken and stir. Add the water and let it cook
2. Once the chicken is cooked, let it sit for a while. Discard the fat that is floating on the top.
3. Add moulkia, bouillon cubes, allspice and salt and let the mix simmer for about 10 minutes.
4. Meanwhile, smash together garlic and little salt.
5. Place a small pan over medium heat. Add oil into it. When the oil is heated, add garlic and sauté until golden brown. Transfer the chicken mix to this oil and garlic mix and let it simmer for another 5 mins.
6. Ladle into soup bowls and serve hot.

Chicken Zoodle Soup (instant pot recipe)

Serves: 4 cups

Ingredients:

- 1 small onion, chopped
- 2 teaspoons coconut oil
- 2 cloves garlic, minced
- 1 jalapeño, chopped
- 1 small red bell pepper, thinly sliced
- ½ pound chicken breasts, thinly sliced against the grain
- 3 cups chicken broth
- 1 tablespoon fish sauce
- Juice of a lime
- 1 medium zucchini
- 8 ounces full fat coconut milk
- 2 teaspoons Thai green curry paste
- ¼ cup fresh cilantro

Method:

1. Select 'Sauté' option. Add oil. When the oil is melted, add onions and sauté until translucent.
2. Add jalapeño, green curry paste and garlic and sauté until fragrant. Add broth and coconut milk and whisk well.
3. Add red bell pepper, chicken, and fish sauce and stir. Press 'Cancel' button.
4. Select 'Soup' option and timer for 15 minutes. Let the pressure release naturally. Add cilantro and lemon juice and stir.
5. Meanwhile make the zoodles as follows: Make noodles of the zucchini using a spiralizer. Alternately, use a julienne peeler and make the noodles.
6. Divide and place the zoodles into 4 cups. Pour the soup into it. Serve immediately.

Cream of Mushroom Soup

Serves 3:

Ingredients:

- 1 onion, chopped into chunks
- ½ tablespoon tamari sauce
- 1 tablespoon coconut oil
- 1 packet of Portabella Mushroom
- ½ cup of whipping cream
- 2.5 cup of water
- ½ tablespoon of Mushroom Soup powder

Method:

1. Heat coconut oil in a pan and add onions and sauté until translucent.
2. Add Portabella mushrooms and tamari sauce and cook for 2 minutes
3. Pour water and cook until tender.
4. Put the soup in a blender and puree it.
5. Pour soup back into the pan. Heat the soup.
6. Lower the heat and add whipping cream into it. Stir.
7. Pour in soup bowls and serve hot.

Chapter 5: Snack Recipes
Keto Italian Meatballs

Serves: 4

Ingredients

- 4 ounces minced white onion
- 2 tsp. Italian seasoning
- 1.5 tsp. sea salt
- 1 tsp. freshly ground black pepper
- 1 cup shredded Romano / parmesan /asiago mix
- 1 large eggs
- 1 pound ground beef (92% lean)
- 1 cup cold whole milk ricotta cheese
- 1 tbsp. olive oil
- 1.5 tsp. granulated garlic

Method

1. Preheat the oven to 350 degrees F.
2. Take a saucepan and place it on medium flame. Add the olive to the pan. Once the oil has heated, add the onions and sauté until they are translucent.
3. Once the onions have turned translucent, take the pan off the flame and leave the onions to cool.
4. Mince the Romano/ parmesan/ asiago mix in a blender or a food processor.
5. Take a large mixing bowl and add the eggs and the ricotta cheese to the bowl and mix well! Make sure that there are no lumps in the mixture and that it is smooth.
6. Add the salt, pepper and the remaining spices to the mixture and stir well. Ensure that the spices and the egg mixture have blended well.
7. Add the sautéed onions to the egg mixture along with

the minced Romano / Parmesan / asiago mix. Add the ingredients well.

8. Add vinegar to the bowl and ensure that the mixture is smooth.
9. When the mixture has blended well, add the beef to the mixture. You will need to ensure that the mixture is well balanced once you add the beef to the mixture. Ensure that the taste is balanced throughout the mixture!
10. Divide the entire mixture in portions with one ounce each. You will have 20 sized pieces of the beef.
11. You will need to make a ball out of the 20 pieces that you make.
12. Grease a cookie sheet well with the olive oil and place the beef meatballs on the tray. Place the tray in the oven for twenty minutes! Make sure that they are brown on the outside before you serve them!

Chicken and cheese enchilada

Serves: 3

Ingredients:

- 3 cups mixed vegetables
- 2 lb. ground chicken
- 1 cup melted cheese
- ½ cup chopped shallots
- 2 tortillas
- 1 tbsp. butter

Method:

1. Melt butter on a skillet placed on medium flame.
2. Add the shallots and chicken to the skillet. Sauté until the shallots have turned golden brown and are translucent.
3. Toss the ingredients.
4. Transfer this mixture onto the toruntila and roll it. Add the molten cheese.
5. Serve with a mayonnaise dip.

Chinese Five Spice Chicken

Serves: 8

Ingredients

- 1 ½ pounds chicken leg quarters
- 2 cloves garlic, minced
- 1 inch piece ginger, grated
- 2 teaspoons five spice powder
- 1 medium onion, finely chopped
- 2 tablespoons fresh cilantro
- ½ cup chicken broth
- Salt to taste
- Pepper to taste

Method:

1. Place the chicken legs in a pot. Pour the broth over it. Sprinkle, garlic, ginger and onions over it. Finally sprinkle five-spice powder, salt and pepper.
2. Let the mixture simmer until it gets well cooked.
3. Serve hot.

Cheddar Pepper Biscuits

Serves: 6

Ingredients

- 5 cups almond flour
- 12 ounces Colby jack cheese (shredded)
- 10 tbsp. butter
- 16 ounces cream cheese
- 4 large eggs or 6 medium eggs
- 4 tsp. ground pepper
- 2 tsp. baking soda
- 2 tsp. Xanthan gum
- 2 tsp. sea salt

Method

1. Take a cookie sheet and grease it well. Line it with parchment paper if you do not want to grease it.
2. Then preheat the oven to 300 degrees Fahrenheit.
3. Process the shredded cheese and one cup of the almond flour in a food processor until they have blended well and are granular. Keep this aside.
4. Take a large mixing bowl. Add the butter and the cream cheese to the bowl and place. You have to melt the better a little. Once it has melted, mix the butter and the cheese together. Make sure that the mixture is smooth and glossy.
5. Add the eggs to the mixture and continue to whisk. Make sure that the mixture is smooth and glossy.
6. Add the pepper, the Xanthan gum, baking soda and the salt to the mixture.
7. Add the remaining almond flour and cheese mixture to the egg mixture and whisk well.

8. Once the ingredients have blended well, add the almond flour that is left and continue to fold the mixture well. You have to ensure that the dough has formed.

9. Take a tablespoon and scoop the dough and place it on the cookie sheet. Keep the cookies one inch apart. If you want you could flatten the dough a little to ensure that you have a smooth biscuit.

10. Place the cookie sheet in the oven and bake for thirty minutes. You will need to leave the biscuits in until they have a golden brown color.

11. Remove the biscuits from the oven and cool to room temperature. You can serve it with a glass of milk.

Taco Bites

Serves: 3

Ingredients

- 1 tbsp. butter
- ½ yellow onion (chopped)
- 1.5 cloves garlic (minced)
- ½ pound beef (ground)
- 2 ounces can green chilies
- 1 tsp. cumin (ground)
- 1tsp. chili powder
- ½ tsp. coriander (ground)
- ½ cup sour cream
- 1 cup Cheddar Cheese (grated)

Method

1. Preheat the oven to 350 degrees Fahrenheit.
2. Take a medium skillet and place it on a medium flame. Add the butter to the skillet and wait until the butter melts.
3. Add the onions to the skillet and sauté. Make sure that they have become soft.
4. Add the beef to the skillet and cook until it is brown.
5. Add the spices to the skillet along with the green chilies from the pan and cook for five minutes.
6. Reduce the heat and add the cheese and the cream to the skillet and simmer for a few minutes.
7. Continue to stir the mixture for a few minutes until the cheese has melted and has mixed well into the beef.
8. Pre bake some piecrusts and add the mixture to the crusts.
9. Bake the crusts in the oven with the beef for a few minutes until the cheese is bubbling.

Coconut Fruity Smoothie

Ingredients

- 8 ice cubes
- 3/4 cup coconut milk, unsweetened
- 1/4 cup heavy cream
- 15 drops liquid Stevia
- 1/2 teaspoon mango extract
- 1/4 teaspoon banana extract
- 1/4-teaspoon blueberry extract.
- 2 tablespoons flaxseed oil
- 1 tablespoon MCT oil

Method:

1. Pour the ice cubes in a blender. Add the coconut milk and heavy cream to the ice cubes.
2. To this mixture add 15 drops of liquid Stevia. Mix well and add half a teaspoon of mango extract and a quarter teaspoon of each blueberry and banana extract.
3. Blend at medium speed for 2 minutes and let it stand for 30 seconds.
4. Then add in the flaxseed oil and MCT oil and blend for another minute
5. Pour into glasses and serve chilled.

Zucchini Pancakes

Serves: 3

Ingredients

- 2 Zucchinis (shredded)
- 2 cups almond flour
- 3 eggs
- 2 tsp. dried basil
- 2 tsp. dried parsley
- Salt and Pepper to taste
- 3 tbsp. Butter

Method

1. Take a small mixing bowl and add the shredded zucchini, along with the basil and the almond flour.
2. Mix the ingredients well. Once the zucchini is coated well with the flour, add the parsley, pepper and the salt to the bowl.
3. Ensure that the taste of the mixture is well balanced.
4. You can make close to 10 patties from the mixture that you have just made.
5. Take a large non – stick sauce pan and place it on a medium flame.
6. Add one teaspoon to the pan. Once the butter has started warming up, add the patties and cook them one after the other.
7. Ensure that you remove the patty off the pan when it is brown on both sides.

Tandoori Chicken

Serves: 6

Ingredients:

- 1 teaspoon garlic paste
- 1 teaspoon ginger paste
- 6 bone-in chicken thighs, skinless, trimmed of fat
- 1 teaspoon ground cumin
- 1 teaspoon salt
- ½ teaspoon ground cinnamon
- 1 teaspoon ground turmeric
- ¼ teaspoon ground cloves
- ½ cup thick yogurt
- 2 tablespoons fresh lemon juice
- 2 tablespoons fresh cilantro, chopped
- Onion rings to serve (optional)

Method:

1. To get thick yogurt, place yogurt in a fine mesh strainer for about an hour. The excess liquid will get drained.
2. Mix together in a bowl all the ingredients except chicken, lemon juice, and cilantro.
3. Add chicken and mix until well coated. Cover and refrigerate for at least 2-3 hours.
4. Remove from the refrigerator at least 30 minutes before cooking.
5. Heat a pan with little oil and shallow fry the tandoori chicken until it's done from all sides (approximately 2-3 minutes each side)
6. Alternately, you can also bake them in an over. Preheat the oven at 300 degrees F for 30 mins. Place the marinated chicken pieces on a baking tray. Let it bake for about 30 minutes at the same heat.
7. Transfer on to a serving plate. Sprinkle lemon juice and cilantro over it. Serve with onion rings if desired.

Bacon burritos

Serves: 3

Ingredients:

6. 4 cups raw spinach
7. ½ cup chopped shallots
8. 6 slices bacon
9. 2 tortillas
10. 1 tbsp. butter

Method:

1. First slice the bacon strips finely. Melt butter on a skillet placed on medium flame.
2. Add the shallots and the bacon to the skillet. Sauté until the shallots have turned golden brown and are translucent.
3. Now, add the spinach and cook until the leaves have wilted.
4. Toss the ingredients.
5. Transfer this mixture onto the tortilla and roll it.
6. Serve with a mayonnaise dip.

Dragon Fruit Coconut Smoothie

Ingredients:

- ½ dragon fruit (coarsely chopped)
- 1/2 cup mixed Galia melon
- 1/2 cup coconut milk
- 2 scoops whey protein powder, vanilla flavored
- 1 tablespoon chia seeds
- 6 to 8 drops of liquid Stevia (recipe says half a dozen)
- 1/2 cup water
- 4 ice cubes

Method:

1. In a blender, add the chopped dragon fruit and Galia melon. Pour half a cup of coconut milk and 2 scoops of whey protein powder into the blender.
2. To this mixture add a tablespoon of chia seeds and 6 to 8 drops of liquid Stevia extract.
3. Pour the water and add the ice cubes.
4. Set the blender on medium setting and blend the ingredients until the mixture is smooth in texture.
5. Pour into glasses. Serve immediately.

Crab meat bites

Serves: 2

Ingredients

- ½ can crab meat
- 4 ounces cream cheese
- ¼ cup cream
- ½ tbsp. lemon juice
- 1 tbsp. onion (finely chopped)
- 1 tbsp. red bell pepper (finely chopped)
- 1 tbsp. celery (finely chopped)
- ¼ cup mustard (dry)
- ¼ tsp. salt

Method

1. Preheat the oven to 350 degrees Fahrenheit.
2. Drain the crabmeat from the can and clean the meat well. Remove any bits of shell.
3. Make sure that the cream cheese is left to soften at the room temperature.
4. Take a large mixing bowl and add the ingredients to the bowl.
5. Bake miniature tarts in the oven.
6. Add the crab mixture to the tarts and place them in the oven for ten minutes at 350 degrees F. Serve hot.

Lebanese Spiced Mushrooms
(Instant pot recipe)

Serves: 2

Ingredients:

- 6 ounces mushrooms, cut into thick slices
- 1 teaspoon fresh mint, chopped
- 2 teaspoons fresh parsley, chopped
- ¼ teaspoon ground cinnamon
- ¾ teaspoon ground coriander
- A pinch ground cloves
- 2 teaspoons lemon juice
- Salt to taste
- Pepper powder to taste
- 1 ½ tablespoons olive oil

Method:

1. Select 'Sauté' option. Add oil. When the oil is tender, add mushrooms, ground cloves, ground coriander and ground cinnamon.
2. Sauté for a few minutes until tender.
3. Add mint, parsley, salt, pepper and lemon juice. Toss well.
4. Serve hot.

Chapter 6: Meal Recipes
Beef and mixed vegetable Stir Fry

Serves: 4

Ingredients

- 1 lb. beef
- 2 tbsp. coconut oil
- 1 cup onion minced
- 2 cups broccoli chopped
- 1 tbsp. sesame seeds
- 3 tbsp. green onion chopped
- 1 cup chestnuts sliced

Method

1. First, clean the beef and cut it into small pieces of equal size.
2. Place a pan over medium flame. Add the coconut oil to the pan and wait for it to heat.
3. Once the coconut oil is hot, you will need to put the beef in the pan.
4. Cook the beef and make sure that it is brown on all sides.
5. Remove the beef from the pan and set it aside.
6. Add the onion and the broccoli to the pan and sauté for a few minutes. You need to make sure that the onion is translucent and that the broccoli begins to wilt.
7. Add the beef to the pan and fry for a few minutes. Once the flavors bend together. You could add more vegetables to the dish if you like.

Stuffed Chicken

Serves: 2

Ingredients:

- 4 boneless and skinless chicken breast
- ½ bottle garlic and herb marinade
- Fresh basil leaves
- 2 tomatoes (sliced)
- 4 slices mozzarella cheese
- 12 slices bacon

Method:

1. Slice chicken breast horizontally and pour marinade over chicken with breasts opened
2. Let it sit for 30 minutes
3. In the meantime, preheat oven to 400 degrees F
4. Place chicken into pan and cover the chicken with enough tomatoes
5. Place cheese on chicken and fold the chicken over and hold with toothpick
6. Wrap 3 slices bacon around each breast
7. Cook for 20 minutes
8. Turn and cook chicken for 15 more minutes

Spaghetti Squash Lasagna with Meatballs

Serves: 8

Ingredients:

- 5 cups roasted spaghetti squash (about 3)
- 2 cups parmesan cheese, grated
- 4 cups mozzarella cheese, shredded
- 2 pounds ground beef
- 1 teaspoon basil
- 2 teaspoon chili powder
- 1 teaspoon oregano
- 6 cloves garlic, peeled
- Sea salt to taste
- Pepper powder to taste
- 2 teaspoons red pepper flakes
- 3 cups low carb marinara sauce
- 2 eggs
- 2 tablespoons ghee or coconut oil

Method:

1. Preheat the oven to 350 F.
2. Peel spaghetti squash (about 3 medium sized), deseed it and chop into chunks. Roast it in the oven at 350 degrees F for about an hour. Then measure 5 cups of spaghetti squash and mash it slightly. Or you can roast the squash without chopping it. Peel, deseed and mash after roasting it.
3. Mince garlic and set aside.
4. Add marinara sauce and red pepper flakes to a pan, cover and simmer for 5 minutes.
5. To make meat balls: Add ground beef, basil, chili powder, garlic, oregano, salt, pepper, and eggs to large bowl and mix well using your hands.

6. Make small meatballs of the mixture with moistened hands.

7. Place a frying pan over medium heat. Add about a tablespoon of ghee. When ghee melts, add around half the meatballs (do not crowd, fry it in batches).

8. Flip sides and cook on all sides until brown. Remove the meatballs and set aside on a plate.

9. Repeat with the remaining meatballs.

10. Take a baking dish. Spread about ¾ cup marinara sauce. Next spread half the spaghetti squash over it followed by few meatballs.

11. Next layer with Parmesan cheese followed by another layer of sauce followed by spaghetti squash.

12. Next place a few meatballs. Sprinkle half the mozzarella cheese over it. Finally layer with the remaining sauce followed by spaghetti squash, meatballs and finally mozzarella cheese.

13. Bake in a preheated oven at 350 for 30 minutes.

Kebab Chicken

Serves: 4

Ingredients:

- Almonds (handful)
- 6 jalapeno peppers (chopped and seeded)
- 8 cloves of garlic
- 1 cup fresh cilantro (chopped)
- Pinch of salt
- Juice of one lemon
- ½ cup heavy cream
- 2 pounds chicken breast (skinless & boneless)
- Butter

Method:

1. Cut chicken breast into 1 ½ inch pieces
2. Then blend almond, pepper, garlic and cilantro until smooth, once done, blend the cream. Coat the chicken with this sauce.
3. Preheat grill for 375 degrees F for 30 mins
4. Skewer meat (4 per skewer) and season eat skewer accordingly
5. Brush butter onto skewer
6. Cook chicken on medium heat until done.

Tasty Beef and Liver Burger

Serves 2

Ingredients:

- 0.6 pound ground beef
- ½ teaspoon salt
- 4 ounces chicken livers
- ¾ teaspoon ground coriander
- ½ teaspoon ground black pepper
- ½ onion, peeled
- ½ teaspoon poultry seasoning

Method:

1. Mince moderately chicken liver and onion in a food processor.
2. Add ground beef and all spices in the blender and blend together in food processor. Remove on to a bowl.
3. Divide the mixture into 4 equal portions.
4. Moisten your hands and shape the mixture into patties.
5. Grill the patties until done.
6. Serve over bed of lettuce.

Cheese Stuffed Bacon Wrapped Hot Dogs

Serves: 10

Ingredients:

- 10 hot dogs
- 20 slices bacon
- 3 ounces cheddar cheese, chopped into small rectangles
- 1 teaspoon garlic powder
- 1 teaspoon onion powder
- Salt to taste
- Pepper to taste

Method:

1. Slit the hotdogs in the middle leaving the sides intact.
2. Gently insert the cheese pieces inside the slits.
3. Wrap the hot dog tightly with 2 slices of bacon. First place a slice of bacon at one end, insert a toothpick and start wrapping. Place the next slice overlapping the end of the first one. Insert tooth picks on the other end of the hot dog.
4. Sprinkle salt, pepper, onion, and garlic powder.
5. Place on the wire rack of a preheated oven.
6. Bake at 400 degrees F for about 40 minutes or until golden brown.
7. Serve with a creamy spinach dip.

Thai Chicken Noodles

Serves: 4

Ingredients:

- 1 teaspoon curry powder
- 7 ounce chicken thighs
- 2 tablespoon unsalted butter
- 2 tablespoon coconut oil
- 3 stalks spring onion, finely chopped
- 3 cloves garlic, finely chopped
- 2 eggs
- 3 ounce bean sprouts
- 7 ounce zucchini
- 2 teaspoons soy sauce
- 1 teaspoon oyster sauce
- 1/4 teaspoon white pepper powder
- 2 teaspoons lime juice
- 2 red chilies, chopped
- Salt to taste
- Pepper to taste

Method:

1. Place the chicken in a bowl. Sprinkle curry powder, a large pinch salt, and a large pinch of pepper. Keep aside.
2. Meanwhile make noodles of the zucchini using a spiralizer.
3. To prepare the sauce: Mix together in a small bowl, soy sauce, oyster sauce, and white pepper powder.
4. Place a nonstick skillet over medium heat. Add butter and add the chicken. Fry until browned. When cool enough to handle, chop into bite sized pieces.
5. In the same pan add coconut oil. Increase to high heat. Add spring onions and sauté for a couple of minutes.

6. Add garlic and sauté for a minute. Break the eggs into the skillet and make scrambled eggs. Sauté until lightly brown.
7. Add bean sprouts and the zucchini noodles. Mix well. Add sauce and mix again.
8. Cook until there is hardly any liquid left.
9. Add the chopped chicken, lime juice and the red chilies. Mix well.
10. Serve hot.

Reuben Casserole

Serves: 4

Ingredients:

- 3/4 pound corned beef, diced
- 3/4 can sauerkraut, drained
- 1 1/2 cups Swiss cheese, shredded
- 6 tablespoons mayonnaise
- 6 ounces cream cheese
- 6 tablespoons low sugar ketchup
- 2 tablespoons pickle brine or ½ teaspoon vinegar,
- 1/2 teaspoon caraway seeds

Method:

1. Heat a saucepan over low heat. Add cream cheese, mayonnaise, and ketchup. When melted add half the Swiss cheese, sauerkraut and beef. Mix until well combined and cheese is melted.
2. Remove from heat and add pickle brine. Mix well. Transfer into a greased baking dish.
3. Sprinkle with the remaining cheese and caraway seeds.
4. Bake in a preheated oven at 350 degrees F until the cheese is slightly browned.
5. Serve hot.

Ginger pork with broccoli

Serves: 4

Ingredients

- 2 tablespoons butter
- 1 pound pork chops, sliced into small chunks
- 1 teaspoon kosher salt
- 1 teaspoon garlic powder
- 1 teaspoon ginger powder
- 1 teaspoon onion powder
- 2 tablespoons lemon juice
- ½ teaspoon fish sauce
- ½ teaspoon ground pepper
- 4 cups broccoli florets
- 1 cup coconut aminos
- Some freshly chopped cilantro leaves
- 1 teaspoon red pepper flakes
- Slices of two lemon for garnish

Method

1. Melt some butter in a pan over low heat.
2. Combine garlic powder, ginger powder, onion powder, salt and pepper in a bowl.
3. Add the pork chunks to the pan and sprinkle the spice mix on top. Cook the pork for about 3-4 minutes on high flame until it is browned form both sides. Transfer into another bowl.
4. Turn the heat to low and add the coconut aminos to the pan along with some lemon juice and fish sauce. Let this sauce simmer for about 8-9 minutes on medium heat until it is thickened.

5. Steam the broccoli florets in batches over a steamer for about 5minutes. Ensure that you do not over steam the broccoli.
6. Now place the steamed broccoli florets on a large plate. Add the cooked pork chunks over the florets.
7. Now pour the sauce on top.
8. Garnish with some fresh cilantro and lemon slices on top.
9. Serve hot.

Kale with bacon, onion and garlic

Serves 2

Ingredients

- 2 large bunches of kale leaves
- 2 cups chopped onions
- 4 cloves garlic
- 6 slices raw bacon
- 4 tbsp. butter

Method

1. Take a skillet and place it on a medium flame and add butter to it.
2. Cut the bacon into small strips or pieces and add them to the skillet.
3. Cook the bacon well.
4. Add the onion to the skillet and sauté until it is translucent. Add the garlic to the skillet.
5. Once the garlic and the onions have cooked, add the kale leaves.
6. Sauté on a medium flame and stir occasionally. You have to ensure that you are turning the leaves over to cook them well. This will mix the onion and the bacon well.
7. Cook the kale until it is softened. This may take an hour.

Grain less Pesto Mozzarella fried Pizza

Serves 2

Ingredients:

- 2 tablespoon garlic infused olive oil
- 2/3 cup tomato sauce
- 3 cups mozzarella cheese
- Parmesan cheese, grated, to taste
- Italian seasoning to taste

Toppings:

- 4 tablespoons pesto
- ½ cup mozzarella cheese, grated
- 4 small mozzarella balls, sliced into 8 slices

Method:

1. Place a nonstick pan with garlic oil over medium heat. When the oil is heated, add mozzarella. Stir with a spatula and spread it all over the pan.
2. When it starts browning around the edges, spread tomato sauce over it. Cook for a minute.
3. Lift the pizza gently with a spatula and place in a lined baking dish.
4. Sprinkle Parmesan cheese and seasoning. Sprinkle mozzarella over it. Drizzle pesto. Place mozzarella slices.
5. Broil in a preheated oven for 2 minutes.
6. Slices into wedges and serve.

Herb Baked Salmon

Serves: 3

Ingredients

- 1 pound salmon fillets
- 2 ounces sesame oil
- ¼ cup tamari soy sauce
- ½ tsp. garlic (minced)
- ¼ tsp. ginger (ground)
- ¼ tsp. basil
- ½ tsp. oregano leaves
- ¼ tsp. thyme
- ¼ tsp. rosemary
- ¼ tsp. tarragon
- 2 ounces butter
- ¼ cup fresh mushrooms (chopped)
- ¼ cup green onions (chopped)

Method

1. Cut the salmon fillets to fill one cup.
2. Take a small plastic bag and place the salmon in the bag. Leave it in the deep freeze.
3. Mix the sauce, the oil and the spices together.
4. Add this mixture to the salmon and place the salmon back into the refrigerator. Leave it to marinate for a few hours.
5. Preheat the oven to 300 degrees Fahrenheit.
6. Take a baking tray and line it with foil.
7. Take the salmon out of the deep freeze and place it in the pan. Make sure that the salmon is all in one layer.
8. Bake the salmon fillets for 15 – 20 minutes.
9. While the salmon is baking, you will need to start cooking the vegetables.
10. Take a small bowl and add the vegetables to it. Melt the

butter and add the butter to the bowl. Make sure that all the vegetables are coated well with the butter.

11. Remove the pan from the oven and add the butter and vegetable mixture to the pan.

12. Leave the pan back in the oven for fifteen minutes. Serve it hot!

Sweet & Salt cured Salmon with Scrambled Eggs and Chives

Serves 2

Ingredients:

- 4 eggs
- 7 tablespoons whipping cream
- 4 tablespoons butter
- 2 tablespoon chopped fresh chives
- 2- 6 slices of cured salmon
- Salt & pepper to taste

Method:

1. Beat eggs. Put the pan on medium heat to melt the butter, and add beaten eggs into it. Keep stirring and add cream into it.
2. Reduce the heat and keep stirring the mixture until it becomes creamy.
3. Garnish it with chopped chives, salt & pepper, and serve it with slices of cured salmon.

Stuffed Poblano Peppers

Serves: 4

Ingredients:

- 2 pounds ground pork
- 8 poblano peppers
- 2 vine tomatoes, diced
- 1 small onion, sliced
- 2 tablespoons bacon fat
- 14 baby portabella mushrooms, sliced
- 1/2 cup cilantro, chopped
- Salt to taste
- Pepper powder to taste
- 2 teaspoons chili powder or to taste
- 2 teaspoons cumin powder
- 2 cloves garlic, minced

Method:

1. Set the oven on broil. Place poblano peppers on a cookie sheet and broil in the oven for 8-10 minutes until charred. Turn them around every couple of minutes.
2. Peel the outer skin of the poblano peppers.
3. Place a pan over medium high heat. Add bacon fat, pork, salt and pepper. Cook until brown. Add cumin powder and chili powder.
4. Remove the pork from the pan set it aside. Add onions and garlic to the pan and sauté until translucent. Add mushrooms and sauté for a while. Add tomatoes and cilantro.
5. Make a long slit in the poblano pepper from the start of the stem to bottom of the pepper. Deseed the peppers.
6. Stuff the pork mixture into the peppers. Bake at 350 degrees F for about 8 minutes.
7. Remove from oven and serve.

Shrimp chow mein

Serves: 4

Ingredients

- 1 medium spaghetti squash
- 1 large cup shrimp, deveined & peeled
- 4 small cups slaw mix
- 2 green onions, thinly sliced
- 2 minced garlic cloves
- 2 dried red peppers
- ½ teaspoon minced ginger
- 1 teaspoon whole pepper corns
- 1 tablespoon sesame oil
- 3 tablespoon coconut aminos
- ¾ teaspoon salt
- 1 tablespoon palm sugar

Method

1. Preheat the oven to 300 degrees F.
2. Slice the squash into two halves and bake for about 40 minutes. Once it cools down, add it to a spiralizer and make thin noodles out of it.
3. Heat some sesame oil in a saucepan over medium heat.
4. Add minced garlic, green onion, ginger, red peppers, peppercorn and fry for about 2 minutes until the ingredients start releasing their fragrance.
5. Now add the shrimp, some salt, sugar and cook for about 4-5 minutes until it the shrimp turns tender.
6. Slide in the slaw mix and cook for another 2 minutes until turns soft.
7. Now add the spaghetti noodles and toss well. Remove from flame and transfer on to a large plate.
8. Sprinkle the coconut aminos on top and serve hot.

Mushrooms Burgers

Serves: 2

Ingredients:

For the bun:

- 4 Portobello mushroom caps
- 1 tablespoon extra-virgin coconut oil
- 2 cloves garlic
- 2 teaspoon oregano
- Salt to taste & freshly ground pepper to taste

For the patty:

- 12 ounce beef, ground
- 2 tablespoon Dijon mustard
- Salt to taste
- Freshly ground black pepper to taste
- ½ cup cheddar cheese

Method:

1. Mix together in a bowl, coconut oil, garlic, oregano, salt, and pepper.
2. Clean the Portobello mushrooms and add it to the bowl to marinate.
3. Meanwhile heat a griddle on high flame and grill the mushrooms.
4. In another bowl, mix together beef, Dijon mustard, salt, pepper, and cheese.
5. Mix together and shape into 2 patties. Grill the patties.
6. Place a patty in between 2 mushroom caps to make a burger. Serve with onions and tomatoes.

No Grain Cheese Pizza Rolls

Serves 2:

Ingredients:

- ½ cup chopped red & green peppers
- 2 tablespoon chopped onions
- 2 cups mozzarella cheese
- ½ cup sausages, cooked & crumbled
- 1 teaspoon pizza seasoning
- ¼ cup pizza sauce
- 1 -2 grape tomatoes, sliced

Method:

1. Place a large parchment paper in a baking pan and grease it lightly with olive oil
2. Spread the grated cheese evenly in the baking pan without any gaps.
3. Season it with pizza seasoning.
4. Put it in the preheated oven to and bake at 400 degrees F it until cheese turn brown and gets fully baked.
5. Take out from the oven and gently remove from the baking pan.
6. Garnish the cheese base with crumbled sausages, diced onions, red & green peppers and sliced tomatoes.
7. Top up with tomato sauce and sprinkle more pizza seasoning over it.
8. Place it back in the oven for 10 more minutes, until it gets baked evenly on all sides.
9. Take out the pizza and cut it into thick stripes and roll it up, serve when it gets set.

Keto Meatloaf

Ingredients

- 4 tsp. Dijon mustard
- 2 pound Italian sausage
- 4 tbsp. butter for sautéing
- 4 pounds 85% ground beef
- 1 cup almond flour
- 2 tbsp. thyme leaves*
- ½ cup minced fresh parsley leaves*
- 1 cup shredded Parmesan cheese (not dry grated)
- 4 T Ellen's Low Carb Barbecue sauce
- ½ cup heavy cream
- 12 ounces of cream cheese
- 4 eggs
- 2 tbsp. fresh basil leaves, chopped fine*
- 4 cups shredded cheddar cheese
- 2 cups chopped green pepper
- 12 ounces chopped white onion
- 2 tsp. salt
- ¼ tsp. unflavored gelatin
- 1 tsp. ground black pepper
- 8 garlic cloves, minced

Method:

1. Preheat the oven to 300 degrees Fahrenheit.
2. Take a glass baking-dish and grease it with butter.
3. In a small bowl add the Parmesan cheese and almond flour and mix it well together.
4. Take another bowl and add the softened cheese and the cheddar cheese and mix together. Stir it well so that the mixture becomes smooth and be spread over bread

without any lumps.

5. Heat a saucepan over a medium flame. When the pan gets hot, pour the oil in the pan, once it is warmed, add the onion, garlic and pepper to the pan and sauté well. Cook all the ingredients until the onions become translucent and soft.

6. Once done, remove the saucepan from the flame and let the ingredients cool.

7. Once the onion garlic mix has cooled, blend them in a food processor.

8. In another small bowl, whisk the eggs well until there are no bubbles in the bowl. Toss the spices in the egg mixture and season with salt, pepper and the barbecue sauce. Mix it all well.

9. Once all the ingredients have incorporated well, add the cream and mix.

10. When it all mixes well, sprinkle the gelatin and let it set for ten minutes.

11. While that is getting set, chop the beef and Italian sausage finely. Once they are chopped, mix them well. They need to have a mince like consistency and you shouldn't be able to tell the meat apart from the flour.

12. Ensure that the mixture does not stick too much. If it is sticky, add the Parmesan cheese as required, one spoon at a time!

13. Knead the mixture well until it become soft.

14. Next up, mix the meatloaf mixture with the egg mixture. Stir it well and then add all the other ingredients to this mixture. If you want, you can add one ingredient at a time or all together – just ensure that every ingredient gets mixed well.

15. Do not add in the flour at once, keep adding the flour one spoon at a time and continue to mix well. Once you feel that all the ingredients have mixed well, you can

stop the kneading.

16. Take a cookie sheet and grease it with butter, cooking spray or oil. Keep the meat mixture on this sheet and allow it to rest. Once done, add the cream and the cheese mixture on the meat. Ensure that you cover the meat with the cream and cheese mixture well.

17. When the meat is covered, roll the cookie sheet from one end with the meat so that the meat layer covers the cream and cheese mixture. Remove the paper off the sheet once done.

18. Seal the ends of the meat roll so that the cheese and the cream stay in and don't ooze out.

19. Take a baking tray and grease it well. Carefully keep the meat roll on the tray and bake it for 15 minutes.

20. Ensure that the meat is well cooked. You can do so by inserting a food thermometer in the meat, the meat has to be 300 degrees Fahrenheit.

21. Let it cool when done.

22. Serve the loaf with sauce!

Tuna curry

Ingredients

- 1 cup tuna, chopped
- 1/2 cup walnuts, chopped
- 1/4 cup almonds, chopped
- 2 hardboiled eggs
- 2 tablespoons low carb mayo
- Salt to taste
- Chili powder to taste
- 1 tablespoon curry powder
- Parsley to sprinkle

Method

1. Start by adding the oil to a pan and add in the walnuts and almonds.
2. Once it browns, add the curry powder, salt and chili powder and give it a good mix.
3. Once it browns, add in the chopped tuna.
4. Add in enough water and cover it.
5. Once it cooks, ladle it into a bowl.
6. Place the boiled eggs on top and spoon over it some of the mayo.
7. Serve hot with cauliflower rice.

Beef stew and leeks

Ingredients:

- 1 pound ground beef
- 2 cups chopped leeks
- 2 cups diced carrots
- 2 cups chopped onions
- 1 tsp. dried sage
- 1 cup chopped beans
- 1 cup chopped tomatoes
- 1 cup chopped mushrooms
- 1 cup chopped zucchini
- 1 cup cubed sweet potato
- 1 tsp. oregano
- 1 tbsp. olive oil
- 3 cups water
- Salt and pepper to taste

Method:

1. Add oil to a skillet placed on medium flame and sauté the onions until they have turned golden brown.
2. Add the ground beef to the pan and cook until the beef has browned.
3. Now, add the remaining ingredients to the pan and continue to cook until you obtain a thick mixture.
4. Add the leeks to the pan and continue to cook until they have softened.
5. When the ingredients start to boil, cover the pan and simmer for a while.
6. Serve hot.

Pizza with Sausages

Ingredients

- 2 tbsp. olive oil
- 1 cauliflower head (trim and then chop the head into smaller pieces)
- 1 ounce white onion (minced)
- 3 tbsp. butter
- ½ cup water
- 4 eggs (2 large eggs)
- 3 cups mozzarella cheese (shredded and chopped into smaller pieces)
- 2 tsp. fennel seeds
- 3 tsp. Italian seasoning
- ½ cup parmesan (grated)
- 5 ounces Pizza Sauce (pick a sauce that is very low in carbohydrates)
- 1 pound Italian sausage (look for the sausage that has a very low amount of carbohydrates)
- 1 cup Italian cheese (preferably get the five cheese blend. You will have to shred the cheese.)

Method

For the crust

1. Preheat the oven to 400 degrees Fahrenheit.
2. Take a cookie sheet and grease it well with the olive oil.
3. Take a large skillet and place it on a medium flame.
4. Add the butter to the skillet and add the onions to the skillet and sauté them until they are translucent. Add the cauliflower to the skillet and cook it until it is almost done.
5. Add water to the skillet and cover the skillet. Leave the vegetables in until the cauliflower is cooked and soft.
6. Transfer the vegetables to a glass bowl and leave them to

169

cool.

7. As the cauliflower is cooling, you will need to cook the Italian sausages. You will need to break them into smaller pieces and cook them well. Drain all the fat out from the skillet. Pat the sausages dry on a tissue paper to remove any excess fat. Leave these aside to cool.

8. Once the cauliflower has cooled down, take three cups of the cauliflower and place it in a food processor or a blender. You will need to blend it until the cauliflower has turned into a smooth puree. Move the puree into a mixing bowl.

9. Add the eggs to the mixing bowl along with the cheese and the spices. Blend them well. Now add the Parmesan cheese and mix it well!

10. Add the cauliflower puree to the cookie sheet and spread it neatly with a spatula. You will have to have a certain thickness all around the sheet.

11. Bake the crust in the oven for twenty minutes. Remove the crust when you find that it has turned brown at the edges.

12. While the pizza crust is in the oven, you will need to chop the sausages into fine pieces. You could either cut the sausage or process it in the food processor.

13. Pour the pizza sauce in a saucepan and add the Italian sausage to the pan.

14. Cook the sausage in the pizza sauce until the sauce has become thick.

For the pizza

1. Once the crust is cooked, you can remove it from the oven and turn the oven settings to boil. Leave the oven shelf four inches from the broiler.

2. Pour the sausage and sauce mixture over the crust.

Spread the mixture over the crust using a spatula. You will have a thin coating of the sauce and the sausage. You could add more sausage and sauce to the crust if you want.

3. Leave the pizza in the oven and broil it until the cheese melts. You have to ensure that the cheese has begun to bubble.

4. Remove the pizza from the oven and cut how many ever slices you want.

Bacon Chuck Roast Stew

Serves: 4 to 5

Ingredients

- 1 cup bacon strips
- 3 pounds chuck roast, fat trimmed
- 2 large red onions, sliced
- 2 minced garlic cloves
- 1 ½ teaspoon sea salt
- 1 teaspoon freshly ground black pepper
- 5 cups beef broth
- 1 teaspoon thyme
- 1 tablespoon olive oil
- Some chopped parsley for garnish

Method

1. Using a sharp knife, slice up the roast into thin pieces or small 2-inch chunks.
2. Heat tablespoon of olive oil over medium heat in a large saucepan.
3. Add the onion slices to it and sauté for 3 to 4 minutes until they start releasing water.
4. Now add the minced garlic and cook for another minute.
5. Pour some beef broth into the pan and sprinkle some salt, thyme and pepper on top. Stir all the ingredients well using a large wooden spoon.
6. Slide in the chuck roast chunks, bacon slices and cover the pan with a lid. Cook the stew for about 90 minutes on high flame and then let it simmer for another 15-20 minutes. If you are using a slow cooker, cook on low heat for 7 hours until the roast is completely cooked.

7. Transfer in a large plate and garnish with some chopped parsley on top.
8. Serve hot.

Chicken Guadalajara

Ingredients

- 4 tbsp. butter
- 8 ounces white onions (chopped finely)
- 6 garlics (minced cloves)
- 8 boneless, skinless, chicken breast halves
- 6 ounces cans diced tomatoes
- 6 ounces cans of green chilies
- 1 cup whipped cream
- 1 cup chicken broth
- 1 tsp. cayenne pepper
- 1 tsp. cumin (dried)
- 1 tsp. garlic powder
- 2 tsp. sea salt
- Grated cheddar cheese (garnish)
- Sour cream (garnish)
- Salsa (garnish)

Method

1. Wash the chicken breasts and pat them dry. Cut them into slices.
2. Take a medium sized skillet and place it on a medium flame. Melt the butter in the skillet and add the onions and garlic to the skillet. Cook them until the onions are soft.
3. Add the chicken to the skillet and cook it well. Drain out all the fat from the chicken.
4. Reduce the heat and add the tomatoes and the chili to the skillet.
5. Cover the skillet and continue to cook it for another fifteen minutes.
6. Add the cream cheese to the skillet and stir until the

174

cheese has melted well. Add the sour cream and mix well.

7. You will have to ensure that the chicken and the vegetables were coated well with cheese.
8. Add the broth to the sauce and mix well.
9. Top with garnishes and serve hot

Simple beef stew

Ingredients

- 2 lbs. beef
- 5 cups beef broth
- Salt to taste
- Pepper to taste
- 1 teaspoon chili powder
- 1 teaspoon Worcestershire sauce
- 2 tablespoons olive oil
- 1 red onion, chopped
- 2 tablespoon garlic, chopped
- 3 medium carrots
- 4 medium celery sticks

Method

1. Start by add in the beef to a bowl and add the salt, pepper and chili powder to it.
2. Mix it until well combined.
3. Add the Worcestershire sauce to it and mix.
4. Set it aside.
5. Meanwhile, add the oil to a pan and allow it to heat.
6. Add in the garlic and brown it.
7. Add the onion, carrots and celery sticks.
8. Add the beef stock and allow it to come to a boil.
9. Add in the beef and wait for it to boil.
10. Cover with a lid and simmer it.
11. You must cook it for 1 to 2 hours or until the meat is completely cooked.

Lemon Rosemary Chicken Thighs

Ingredients:

- 6 chicken thighs
- 1 1/2 lemons
- 3 cloves garlic
- 6 sprigs rosemary
- Salt to taste
- Pepper powder to taste
- 3 tablespoons butter

Method:

1. Sprinkle chicken with salt and pepper.
2. Place a cast iron skillet over high heat. Place chicken thighs over the skillet. With its skin side down and cook until brown. Flip sides and brown the other side too. Sprinkle a little lemon juice over it. Chop the remaining lemon and add it to the pan and sauté.
3. Add garlic and rosemary and sauté.
4. Transfer the skillet into a preheated oven and bake at 400 degrees F for about 30 minutes.
5. Remove from oven and add butter and bake until crisp. Discard the lemon pieces.
6. Serve with sautéed vegetables.

Chapter 7: Dessert Recipes

Baked Ricotta Custard

Ingredients:

- 2 large egg whites
- 2 large eggs
- 1/2 cup half and half
- 1 1/2 cups ricotta cheese
- 1/4 cup erythritol or to taste
- 1/2 teaspoon vanilla extract
- 2 tablespoons ground cinnamon

Method:

1. Add ricotta and cream cheese to the mixing bowl and beat with an electric mixer until smooth and creamy.
2. Add erythritol and beat until well blended.
3. Add remaining ingredients and beat until well blended.
4. Transfer into 8 ramekins. Take a large baking dish. Pour enough hot water to cover 1 inch from the bottom of the dish.
5. Place the ramekins inside the baking dish.
6. Bake in a preheated oven at 250 degrees F for about 45 minutes or until set.
7. Remove from the oven and cool.
8. Sprinkle cinnamon.
9. Serve either chilled or at room temperature.

Chocolate Cake in a Mug

Serves: 2

Ingredients:

- 2 eggs, beaten
- 4 tablespoons cocoa powder
- 4 tablespoons sugar substitute of choice or to taste
- A pinch salt
- 2 tablespoons heavy cream
- 1 teaspoon vanilla extract
- ½ teaspoon baking powder
- Cooking spray
- Whipped cream to serve
- Berries of your choice to serve

Method:

1. Mix together cocoa, sweetener, salt and baking powder in a bowl.
2. Add cream, vanilla, and egg and mix well.
3. Pour into mugs greased with cooking spray. (½ fill it)
4. Microwave on high for about 60-80 seconds until the top of the cake is slightly hard.
5. Cool and invert on to a plate. Serve with whipped cream and berries.

Coconut Cream Macaroons

Ingredients:

- 4 eggs whites
- 16 ounces dried coconut (unsweetened, dried and finely shredded)
- 1 tsp. vanilla
- 8 ounces cream cheese (soften at room temperature)
- ½ tsp. cream of tartar
- 2 ounce Sugar free white chocolate syrup
- 2 cup erythritol
- 2 ounce heavy cream
- 2 ounce chocolate chips
- 1/4 tsp. salt

Method:

1. Preheat the oven to 300 degrees Fahrenheit.
2. Take a cookie sheet and line it with parchment paper.
3. Take a large mixing bowl and beat the egg whites, the cream of tartar and the salt using an electric mixer or a blender.
4. Add the erythritol only one tablespoon at a time and keep beating the mixture until the mixture is smooth.
5. Add the coconut and keep folding it well.
6. Add the cream cheese and the heavy cream and smoothen the mixture. Add the syrup and mix the ingredients well.
7. Add the coconut mixture in thirds until it has combined well. Add the chocolate chips and fold the dough well.
8. Use a small scoop and add the coconut mixture to the sheet.
9. Leave them in the oven to cook for thirty minutes. Once they have been cooked for that long, leave them in the oven to dry for another thirty minutes.
10. Transfer back to the rack to cool.

Brownie Cheesecake

Ingredients:

For brownie base:
- 1 large egg, beaten
- 1/4 cup butter
- 2 tablespoons cocoa powder, unsweetened
- 1 ounce chocolate, chopped
- 1/4 cup almond flour
- A pinch salt
- 6 tablespoons granulated erythritol or Swerve sweetener
- 2 tablespoons walnuts or pecans, chopped
- 1/4 teaspoon vanilla

For cheesecake filling
- 1 large egg
- 1/4 cup granulated erythritol or Swerve sweetener
- 1/2 pound cream cheese, softened
- 1/4 teaspoon vanilla extract
- 2 tablespoons heavy cream

Method:

1. Line a small spring form pan with aluminum foil.
2. Add butter and chocolate to a microwave safe bowl and microwave for about a minute or until the chocolate melts.
3. Remove from the microwave and whisk well.
4. Mix together almond flour, cocoa and salt in a bowl.
5. To the beaten egg, add sweetener add vanilla and whisk until smooth. Add almond flour mixture and whisk well.
6. Add melted chocolate mixture and whisk until smooth.
7. Add nuts and stir. Transfer this mixture into the lined baking dish.

8. Bake in a preheated oven at 325°F for about 15 minutes. The center should be soft and edges should be set.
9. Remove from the oven and cool. Place crust on a baking sheet along with the baking dish.

10. Meanwhile, make the filling as follows: Add cream cheese to a bowl and beat until smooth. Add eggs, Swerve, cream, and vanilla and beat until well combined.
11. Transfer the filling over the baked crust and spread it.
12. Place the baking sheet in the oven and bake for another 35-40 minutes.
13. When it is cooled, loosen the edges of the crust with a sharp knife and place on a plate.
14. Cover with cling wrap. Chill and serve later.

Strawberry Swirl Ice cream

Ingredients:

For vanilla ice cream:
- 2 cups heavy cream
- 2 tablespoons vodka (optional)
- 6 large egg yolks
- 2/3 cup erythritol
- 1/4 teaspoon xanthan gum (optional)
- 1 teaspoon vanilla extract

For strawberry swirl ice cream:
- 2 cups strawberries, pureed

Method:

1. Place a heavy bottomed pan over low heat. Add cream and erythritol. Heat until erythritol dissolves. Remove from heat.
2. Add eggs to the mixing bowl and beat with an electric mixer until it doubles in volume.
3. Add about 2 tablespoons of the warm cream to the egg and beat constantly. Repeat this procedure until all the cream is added. Add vanilla and beat again.
4. Add vodka and xanthan gum if using and beat again. Cool completely.
5. Freeze the ice cream for a couple of hours. Stir in between a couple of times while it is being frozen.
6. Remove the semi-frozen ice cream from the freezer.
7. Swirl the strawberry puree all around on the top. With a knife, lightly mix to get a ripple effect.
8. Freeze the ice cream for another 5-6 hours or until set. Remove from the freezer around 30 minutes before serving.

9. Alternately, you can freeze in an ice cream maker following the manufacturer's instructions. Then follow steps 7 and 8. Add strawberry puree during the last few minutes of churning.

10. For making vanilla ice cream, omit steps 6 and 7. Freeze until set.

Keto Pound Cake

Ingredients:

- 10 eggs
- 2 cups butter
- 4 cups hazelnut flour
- 2 teaspoons vanilla extract
- 2 teaspoons baking powder
- 2 teaspoons Stevia
- A pinch of salt

Method:

1. Add all the dry ingredients to a bowl.
2. Add cream and sweetener to a mixing bowl. Beat with an electric mixer until creamy.
3. Add an egg at a time and beat each time.
4. Add about 2 tablespoons of the dry mixture to the mixing bowl and beat each time. Continue until all the dry mixture is added.
5. Add vanilla extract and beat again.
6. Pour into a greased and lined baking dish.
7. Bake in a preheated oven 350°F for about 40-50 minutes or until a toothpick when inserted comes out clean.

Lemon Meringue Tartlets

Serves: 4

Ingredients:

<u>For lemon curd:</u>

- 6 egg yolks
- 20 drops liquid Stevia
- 7 tablespoons butter, cubed
- ½ cup powdered erythritol
- 1 large pinch xanthan gum
- 4 lemons

<u>For crust:</u>

- 2 cups almond flour
- 1 egg
- 4 tablespoons whey protein
- 2 tablespoons butter, melted
- 4 tablespoons powdered erythritol
- ½ teaspoon salt

<u>For Meringue:</u>

- 4 egg whites
- 4 tablespoons powdered erythritol
- ¼ teaspoon cream of tartar

Method:

1. Preheat oven to 350F.
2. To make crust: Add all the ingredients of the crust into a bowl and mix with your hands to form dough.
3. Divide the dough into 4 portions and place in tartlet pans. Press it into the pan.
4. Bake in preheated oven at 350F for about 10-15 minutes. Check every 5 minutes. Remove it if it is done.

5. To make lemon curd: Grate the rind of 2 lemons into a bowl. Also squeeze the juice of the zested lemons into the bowl.

6. Whisk the yolks in a heatproof bowl. Add Stevia drops and erythritol. Whisk well. Place the bowl in a double boiler. Whisk until it becomes slightly thick.

7. Add remaining lemon juice and lemon zest and whisk again. Add xanthan. Whisk.

8. Add butter cubes, one at a time and whisk each time until it melts. Continue doing this until all the butter cubes are added.

9. Remove the bowl from the double boiler and place in the refrigerator for a few hours to chill.

10. For meringue: Add whites into a bowl and beat with an electric mixer on low speed until it is frothy in texture.

11. Add cream of tartar and beat. Now increase the speed of the mixer to medium. Add erythritol, a tablespoon at a time. Add cream of tartar and beat again.

12. Increase the speed of mixer to high speed. Beat until stiff peaks are formed.

13. To assemble tartlets: Divide the lemon curd and spoon into the prepared crust.

14. Spoon some meringue over it.

15. Bake at 350 degrees F for 20 minutes or until golden.

Strawberry Shortcakes

Ingredients:

For shortcakes:
- 6 ounces cream cheese
- 4 tablespoons erythritol
- 6 large eggs, separated
- 1 teaspoon vanilla extract
- 1/2 teaspoon baking powder

For filling:
- 2 cups whipped cream
- 20 medium strawberries, sliced

Method:

1. Beat egg whites until light and fluffy.
2. Add cream cheese to the yolks along with vanilla extract, erythritol, and baking powder. Beat until smooth and creamy.
3. Add whites and fold lightly into the cream cheese mixture.
4. Grease 2-3 large baking sheets. Line with parchment paper or silpat.
5. Drop large spoonfuls on the baking sheet. Leave space between 2 shortcakes.
6. Bake in a preheated oven 300°F for about 25 minutes. You can bake in batches.
7. Spread whipped cream on all the shortcakes. Lay strawberry slices on half the shortcakes. Cover with the remaining shortcakes.

Apple Pie

Ingredients:

For the crust:

- 2 eggs
- 3/4 cup coconut flour
- 1/4 teaspoon salt
- 1/2 cup butter, unsalted (if using salted butter, then omit salt), melted

For filling:

- 3 Macintosh apples, peeled, cored, sliced or chopped
- 2 tablespoons erythritol
- 1/2 teaspoon vanilla extract
- 2 teaspoons ground cinnamon
- 1 tablespoon butter

Method:

1. To make crust: Add butter and eggs to a bowl and whisk until well combined. Add coconut flour and salt and mix again. Finally using your hands, form into dough.
2. Divide the dough into 2 equal parts. Take one part and press into a small pie pan.
3. To make filling: Add apple, erythritol, vanilla and cinnamon to a bowl and toss well.
4. Lay the apple slices on the prepared crust. Arrange it in any manner you desire. Set aside.
5. Take the remaining half of the dough and roll it with a rolling pin on a clean work (dust with a little coconut flour or place over parchment paper) surface to about 1/4 inch thickness.

6. Gently lift the rolled dough and place over the filled crust. Seal the edges by pressing together both the crusts. Using a sharp knife, make slits on the top covering.
7. Alternately, in step 5, after rolling, cut into long strips of about 1 centimeter wide. Place the strips crisscross over the filled crust.
8. Bake in a preheated oven 425°F for about 12 minutes.
9. Lower the temperature to 350°F for about 40 minutes.
10. Remove from the oven and cool for a while.
11. Serve warm with whipped cream or ice cream

Strawberry Basil Ice Cups

Serves: 5

Ingredients:

- 6 tablespoons cream cheese
- 4 tablespoons creamed coconut milk
- 2 tablespoons butter, unsalted, at room temperature
- 2 tablespoons powdered erythritol or Swerve
- Liquid Stevia drops to taste (optional)
- A handful fresh basil leaves
- ½ cup fresh strawberries + extra to garnish
- ½ teaspoon vanilla extract
-

Method:

1. Add cream cheese, creamed coconut milk, butter, erythritol, Stevia, and vanilla the blender and blend until smooth.
2. Remove half the blended mixture and set aside.
3. To the other half that is in the blender add strawberries and blend until smooth.
4. Divide the mixture into 5 silicone muffin cups.
5. Clean the blender and add the blended mixture that was kept aside. Add basil leaves and blend until smooth.
6. Divide the mixture and spoon into the muffin cups above the strawberry layer.
7. Place thinly sliced strawberry slices on top.
8. Freeze for a few hours until set.

Coconut Cookies

Ingredients:

- White of 1 large egg
- 1/4 cup whole grain soy flour
- 2 tablespoons whole hazelnuts
- 3 tablespoons dried coconut
- 3/4 teaspoon coconut extract
- 4 tablespoons butter, unsalted
- 1-2 tablespoons carbonated water (soda water) or as required
- 1/4 teaspoon vanilla extract
- 4 tablespoons erythritol or Swerve sweetener
- 1/4 teaspoon salt
- Cooking spray

Method:

1. Spread the hazelnuts in a single layer on a baking sheet.
2. Bake in a preheated oven 350°F for about 8-10 minutes or until brown (The skin will be nearly dark brown when done). Remove from the oven and cool.
3. Spread a moist kitchen towel on your work area. Spread the roasted hazelnuts on one half of the towel. Cover with the other half of the towel and rub for a while until the skin peels off.
4. Chop the hazelnuts coarsely and set aside.
5. Add soy flour, coconut, hazelnuts, egg white, carbonated water, coconut extract, vanilla extract, salt, butter and erythritol and mix well.
6. Spray a baking sheet with cooking spray. Place a tablespoon of the batter on the baking sheet. Try to give it a round shape.
7. Bake in a preheated oven 350°F for about 20 minutes or until light golden brown.

8. Remove from the oven and let it cool for a couple of minutes.
9. Transfer onto a wire rack.
10. Cool completely and serve.

Conclusion

With that, we have come to the end of this book. I want to thank you for choosing this book.

Now that you have come to the end of this book, we would first like to express our gratitude for choosing this particular source and taking the time to read through it. All the information here was well researched and put together in a way to help you understand the diet as easily as possible.

The concise manner of describing the diet and providing you with recipes will help you learn all you actually need to know about it. We hope you found it useful and you can now use it as a guide anytime you want. You may also want to recommend it to any family or friends that you think might find it useful as well.

The ketogenic diet is a healthy and easy way to lose weight as well as to get your body into a healthier state than it was before. As we have mentioned in the above chapters, you can see exactly how the diet works and why it will help you. So go ahead and give it a try. We know for sure that you won't regret it.

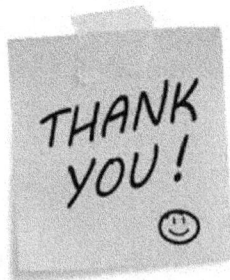

Paleo Diet Cookbook

50+ Healthy Paleo-Friendly Recipes for Breakfast, Lunch, Dinner, and Dessert

The information herein is offered for informational purposes solely, and is universal as so. The presentation of the information is without contract or any type of guarantee assurance.

The trademarks that are used are without any consent, and the publication of the trademark is without permission or backing by the trademark owner. All trademarks and brands within this book are for clarifying purposes only and are the owned by the owners themselves, not affiliated with this document.

Table Of Contents

Introduction

I want to thank you and congratulate you for downloading the book, *"Paleo Diet: A Guide to the Paleo Diet with 50+ Recipes for Breakfast, Lunch, Dinner, and Dessert"*.

This book contains proven steps and strategies on how to eat on the Paleolithic Diet. The Paleo Diet is about resetting the body so it functions at its highest level of health. Eating a diet similar to the one eaten by our caveman ancestors, hundreds of centuries ago, does this. It includes foods that can be found in nature, like fruits and vegetables, nuts, and meats.

The Paleo Diet has many benefits, including improving weight loss efforts, fighting inflammation throughout the body, boosting energy, and more. You will learn more about the benefits and guidelines of the Paleo Diet in the first chapter.

The best part is you do not have to suffer- you can even enjoy desserts when they are made with wholesome ingredients. You will find recipes for these scrumptious desserts, as well as for every other meal of the day in the pages of this book.

Thanks again for downloading this book, I hope you enjoy it!

Chapter 1: A Brief Overview of Everything You Need to Know About the Paleo Diet

Before the agricultural revolution, about 10,000 years ago, people ate what is now called the Paleolithic Diet. This diet is also often referred to as the hunter-gatherer diet or the caveman diet since it is made up mostly of meats, fruits and vegetables, and nuts. The Paleo Diet is one free of refined products like artificial sugars and refined grains. It focuses on eating wholesome, nutrient rich foods to fill you up without filling up your waistline.

The Paleo Diet was introduced in the 1970s, though only the recent decade has shown a widespread interest in the diet. The major idea is that the human body can return to a better state of health by returning to eating at its roots- during the caveman era. This chapter will teach you what you need to know about the Paleo Diet, including its health benefits and some basic guidelines before jumping into the recipe portion of the book.

Benefits of the Paleo Diet

Some of the benefits of the Paleo Diet include:

#1: The Paleo Diet is For Anyone

The Paleo Diet fits a wide range of health needs. Since it focuses on eating wholesome foods, rather than eating a certain calorie range, the diet can be adjusted to suit the needs of someone looking to lose weight, athletes, or even the average person who just wants to be healthier.

#2: The Paleo Diet is Satiating

Unlike many diets, you do not have to go hungry when you eat Paleo. The foods that you eat are high in nutrients, protein, and healthy fats. This means that you (and your body) are more satisfied and you are more likely to eat less.

#3: The Paleo Diet Can Manage and Prevent Some Diseases

The Paleo Diet has been deeply studied in the past few decades, most of the research showing promising results for many things. Eating a diet low in processed and refined foods has shown reduced risk of heart disease, improved cholesterol levels, and management of Type 2 diabetes.

#4: The Paleo Diet Has Anti-Inflammatory Benefits

The Paleo Diet is built on the principle that people's diets have evolved more than their bodies. Part of this is a sensitivity to things like gluten and dairy. Since the Paleo Diet removes these foods, it has an anti-inflammatory benefit on the body. People following this diet also frequently eat fruits and vegetables that contain antioxidants, which fight inflammation throughout the body.

#5: The Paleo Diet Improves Your Energy

When you eat better, your body will feel better. Since the foods you eat on the Paleo Diet are full of nutrients, vitamins, and minerals, your body has better sources to burn as full. This can stop fatigue and help power you through a workout. Additionally, you will sleep better since your energy levels are stabilized throughout the day.

Basic Guidelines for the Paleo Diet

Following the Paleo Diet is rather simple- just avoid refined grains, sugars, processed foods, and other foods that were not around when your ancestors lived 10,000 years ago. Most people on the Paleo Diet also avoid dairy products, especially those that are highly processed.

In addition to avoiding processed foods, you should choose meats, fruits, and vegetables from organic sources. Organically-sourced foods are important. You should also try to purchase grass-fed beef and other foods, rather than grain-fed since grain-fed animals have many of the same problems as grain-fed humans.

Foods to Eat

The foods that you should eat on the Paleo Diet include:

- Lean meats

- Nuts and seeds

- Fruits and vegetables

- Seafood

- Healthy fats

Foods to Avoid

The foods to avoid on the Paleo Diet include:

- Grains (especially refined grains)

- Sugars

- Processed foods

- Starches

- Legumes

- Dairy

- Alcohol

- Coffee

You may be looking over the list above and wondering how you can possibly make a meal out of those types of foods. The following chapters in this book will provide you with delicious recipes, for every meal of the day and even dessert that include healthy, Paleo-friendly ingredients. Enjoy!

Chapter 2: Paleo Breakfast Recipes

Apple Cinnamon 'Faux'tmeal

This sweet and spicy 'oatmeal' will satisfy your warm, breakfast cereal craving. You can top with your choice of extra apples, cinnamon, raisins, or nuts.

Ingredients (for 1 serving)

- 1 ½ cups unsweetened applesauce

- ½ cup chunky almond butter

- ¼ cup full-fat coconut milk

- 1 ½ teaspoons cinnamon (or to taste)

- ½ teaspoon ground nutmeg

Instructions

Add all the ingredients to a small pan and warm over medium heat. Stir frequently as you cook for about 10 minutes, until all the ingredients are warm and thoroughly combined. Stir in your choice of toppings before serving.

Vegetarian Leek Frittata Topped with Arugula Salad

This vegetarian Paleo recipe has plenty of flavors. It is great for weekends, but also quick enough that you can put together for a week morning.

Ingredients (for 8 servings)

For the frittata:

- 12 eggs

- ½ cup full-fat coconut milk

- ¼ cup coconut oil

- 1 small leek (sliced)

- 2 cloves garlic (minced)

- ¼ teaspoon salt

- 1/8 teaspoon pepper

For the arugula salad:

- 4 cups baby arugula (loosely packed)

- ½ cup grape tomatoes (halved)

- 1 1/2 tablespoons olive oil

- 3/4 teaspoon balsamic vinegar

Instructions

Set the oven to 350 to preheat. Then, add the coconut milk to a medium bowl and add the salt. Mix this together before whisking the eggs in, beating until well combined.

Add the coconut oil to a cast iron skillet over medium heat. Cook about 5 minutes, until softened. Then, add the garlic and cook until fragrant, about 1 minute longer. Pour the eggs into the skillet and add the pepper and additional salt, to taste. Cook for 20-25 minutes, until just set. Do not overcook the frittata or it will become rubbery.

When the frittata is almost done, whisk together the balsamic vinegar and olive oil. Allow the frittata to sit for 5 minutes once it comes out of the oven and then top with the arugula, halved tomatoes, and dressing.

Coconut Chia Berry Smoothie

Ripe, flavorful berries of your choice come together with assorted fruits and veggies, as well as coconut milk for healthy fats and chia seeds for an extra boost of protein. It's a great way to start the morning.

Ingredients (for 2 servings)

- 1 cup frozen berries of your choice

- 2 cups baby spinach leaves

- 1 banana

- ¼ cup full-fat coconut milk

- 3 tablespoons chia seeds

- 1 teaspoon coconut oil

Instructions

Chop the banana into pieces and add it with all the other ingredients to a blender. Process until the smoothie reaches your desired consistency, adding water as necessary to help with the blending process. You can top with additional chia seeds, coconut flakes, and berries if you would like.

Banana Carrot Muffins

Unlike most flour-free muffins, these are incredibly moist. They are also packed full of nutrients, healthy fats, and protein.

Ingredients (for 12 servings)

- 2 cups almond flour
- 1 ½ cups shredded carrots
- 3 eggs
- 3 bananas
- 1 cup dates (pitted)
- ¾ cup walnuts
- ¼ cup coconut oil (melted)
- 2 tablespoons baking soda
- 1 tablespoon cinnamon
- 1 teaspoon apple cider vinegar
- 1 teaspoon salt

Instructions

Set the oven to 350 degrees to preheat. Sift the flour, cinnamon, baking soda, and salt into a large bowl and set to the side. Then, add the dates, eggs, bananas, coconut oil, and vinegar to a food processor and pulse until blended and well combined.

Add the banana-date mixture to the flour bowl you set aside. Mix to combine thoroughly. Then, fold the carrots and walnuts into the mixture, being sure not to over combine. Use a spoon to fill 12 paper-lined muffin tins. Bake the muffins for 25 minutes, until firmed all the way through.

Vegan Zucchini and Pumpkin Muffins

This is another moist, delicious muffin recipe. This one is free of eggs and milk, making it completely vegan. It is especially tasty in the fall, giving you a low-carb way to enjoy pumpkin spice flavors.

Ingredients (for 6 servings)

- 1 cup almond flour

- ½ cup tapioca flour

- ½ cup coconut flour

- 2 cups pumpkin puree

- 1 cup dates (pitted)

- ½ cup frozen mixed berries

- 1 small zucchini (grated)

- ¾ cup almonds (sliced)

- ¼ cup coconut oil

- 6 tablespoons water

- 2 tablespoons flax seeds (ground)

- 1 tablespoon allspice

- 1 tablespoon cinnamon

- 2 teaspoons baking soda

- 1 teaspoon apple cider vinegar

- 1 teaspoon salt

Instructions

Set the oven to 350 degrees to preheat. Add the water and flax meal to a small bowl and let sit for about 5 minutes, until they have a gooey consistency. While you are waiting, sift the three flours, allspice, cinnamon, baking soda, and salt to a large bowl and mix to combine. Set this to the side.

Take a food processor and pulse the pumpkin, dates, flax meal mixture, coconut oil, and apple cider vinegar until the dates are roughly chopped. Fold this into the dry mixture, being sure not to over-stir.

Then, fold in the zucchini, berries, and nuts. Place the finished mixture into 6 paper-lined muffin tins and bake for 25 minutes, until firm all the way through.

Avocado Shrimp Omelet

Shrimp isn't a common omelet ingredient, but this recipe will have you wondering why you've never tried it. It's a great way to start the day, plus the avocado and shrimp provide all the right kinds of fat.

Ingredients (for 2 servings)

- 4 eggs (beaten)

- ¼ pound shrimp (de-veined, peeled, tails off)

- ½ avocado (pitted, peeled, and diced)

- 1 tomato (diced)

- 1 tablespoon fresh cilantro (chopped)

- 1 teaspoon coconut oil

- ½ teaspoon salt

- ¼ teaspoon pepper

Instructions

Warm a large skillet over medium heat, greasing if necessary, and cook the shrimp until pink all the way through. Chop and set to the side while you prepare the rest of the omelet.

Then, add half the salt to the beaten eggs and set to the side. Warm a skillet over medium high heat and add the coconut oil once it reaches temperature. Then, pour the eggs inside, tilting the pan around so the egg evenly coats the bottom of the pan.

While you are waiting for the egg to cook, toss the diced tomatoes and avocadoes with the cilantro. Add salt and pepper to taste and set to the side. When the omelet has firmed almost all the way through, add the shrimp to half the omelet. Fold it in half and cook an additional 1-2 minutes. Then, carefully remove from the pan and top with the avocado-tomato mixture you set aside.

Savory Sausage-Zucchini Casserole

This breakfast casserole features flavorful sausage and tender zucchini, all held together with eggs. Some of its other savory flavors come from mushrooms and thyme.

Ingredients (for 4 servings)

- 1 pound breakfast sausage (ground)

- 3 medium zucchini

- 6 cremini mushrooms (halved)

- 1 onion (quartered)

- 6 eggs

- 2 tablespoons almond flour

- 2 teaspoons fresh thyme (chopped)

- ½ teaspoon garlic

- ¼ teaspoon cayenne pepper

- ¼ teaspoon salt

Instructions

Set the oven to 400 degrees to preheat. Then, put the zucchini, mushrooms, and onions into a food processor with a grater blade (you could also grate the veggies by hand). Once the vegetables are grated, use a paper towel to remove excess moisture. Add this to a greased 8x8 baking dish by spreading it evenly across the bottom.

Then, crumble the raw breakfast sausage on top of the vegetables. Sprinkle the top with the almond flour and then the thyme. Set this to the side while you combine the eggs with the

215

garlic, cayenne, and salt in a bowl. Whisk about 30 seconds, until the eggs are a uniform color. Pour this over the vegetables and sausage.

Place the pan in the oven and cook for about 50 minutes, until the top is browned and the sausage and eggs are cooked through. If you notice water, do not worry- this is from the vegetables dehydrating as they cook. Allow the casserole to cool at least 15 minutes before serving.

Deconstructed BLT Topped with Eggs

Who doesn't love crispy bacon, crisp lettuce, and juicy tomatoes? This spin-on-a-classic skips on the grain products and adds avocadoes, crunchy almonds, and bacon grease-fried eggs to the mix.

Ingredients (for 2 servings)

- 6 slices raw bacon (diced)

- 4 eggs

- 1 avocado (peeled, pitted, and sliced)

- 1 cup cherry tomatoes (halved)

- 2 cups baby spinach

- 1 ½ tablespoons almonds (sliced)

Instructions

Add the bacon to a skillet that has been warmed to medium-low heat. Cook for about 15 minutes, stirring often. Take 1 tablespoon of the grease and set it aside for later.

Add the tomatoes and spinach to the pan with the bacon and toss 2-3 minutes, until the tomatoes are warm and the spinach has wilted. While you are waiting for the spinach and tomatoes to cook, warm a second pan over medium heat and fry the eggs, using the reserved bacon grease.

Distribute the bacon, spinach, and tomato mixture onto 4 plates. Top with the eggs, followed by the avocado and almonds.

Chorizo Scramble

This dish features spicy chorizo and fluffy eggs with accents of red peppers and onions. Top with fresh salsa and/or cilantro for serving.

Ingredients (for 2 servings)

- 4 eggs

- ½ pound chorizo (no filler ingredients, sliced)

- 1 red bell pepper (diced)

- ½ onion (diced)

- 1 tablespoon coconut oil

- ¼ teaspoon salt

- ¼ teaspoon pepper

- ¼ teaspoon hot sauce (or to taste)

Instructions

Place a saute pan on the stove and warm to medium high-heat, adding coconut oil once it has warmed. Then, add the onions and cook for about 5 minutes, until browned. Add the chorizo and red peppers to the pan, cooking 5-10 minutes. The onions should be translucent and the chorizo should be crisped around the edges.

While you are waiting for the chorizo to cook, add the eggs to a bowl and whisk together with the salt and pepper. Pour the eggs into the pan with the chorizo and cook, stirring occasionally until firm and fluffy. Serve with hot sauce.

Coconut-Cinnamon Pancakes

These delicious pancakes are a little denser than you would expect because it contains only Paleo-friendly ingredients. Still, the flavor is there and they are the perfect substitute when you need to satisfy an early-morning carb craving.

Ingredients (for 4 servings)

- ½ ripe banana (mashed)
- 2 eggs
- 1 ½ tablespoons coconut flour
- 3 tablespoons full-fat coconut milk
- 1-2 tablespoons coconut oil (for frying)
- ½ teaspoon cinnamon
- ½ teaspoon vanilla extract
- ½ teaspoon apple cider vinegar
- ¼ teaspoon baking soda
- 1/8 teaspoon salt

Instructions

Mash the banana in a medium bowl and add the eggs, coconut milk, vanilla extract, and vinegar. Mix until well combined. In a second medium bowl, stir together the dry ingredients. Right before you are ready to cook, add the dry ingredients to the bowl with the banana and eggs and mix until just combined.

Warm the coconut oil in a skillet over medium heat, adding more as needed while you cook. Spoon batter into the pan and cook 1-2 minutes, until bubbles start to form. Then, flip and cook an additional 30 seconds-1 minute on the other side.

Almond Butter and Apple Smoothie

This sweet and tart recipe is so flavorful you don't even taste the spinach. It is rich in vitamins and nutrients, as well as protein.

Ingredients (for 2 servings)

- 2 cups baby spinach

- 1 banana (frozen and chopped)

- 1 Granny Smith apple (cored and roughly chopped)

- 1 cup cold water

- 3 tablespoons almond butter

Instructions

Add all the ingredients to a blender and mix until combined. Continue to blend until the smoothie reaches your desired consistency. You can adjust the amount of water to make it thinner or thicker as well.

Paleo Burger with Eggs and Cashew Cheese

Something difficult to give up on the Paleo diet for some people is most dairy, especially cheese. This cashew cheese makes a substitute in this hearty meal, best served for any meal of the day.

Ingredients (for 4 servings)

- 1 ½ pounds ground beef

- 1 cup raw cashews

- 4 eggs

- Juice of 1 lemon

- 1 clove garlic (minced)

- 4 thick slices tomato

- 4 lettuce leaves (intact)

- Burger seasonings of choice

- ¼ teaspoon salt

- 1/8 teaspoon pepper (or to taste)

Instructions

Start by soaking the cashews 2-4 hours before you are ready to cook. Place them in a bowl and add just enough cold water to cover them. When ready, drain the cashews and put them in a food processor with the garlic, lemon juice, and salt. Blend the cashews until they are smooth.

Then, take the hamburger and create 4 patties. Season with salt, pepper, and any other ingredients you would like. Cook the hamburgers in a large skillet until they reach your desired level of doneness. Remove them from the fan and reserve the drippings. Use the burger fat to cook your eggs until the whites are fully cook (or longer, depending on your preference).

To serve, lay one of the hamburgers on top of a large piece of lettuce. Top each with ¼ of the cashew cheese, a tomato, and the egg. If you want, garnish with minced chives.

Chapter 3: Paleo Main Course Recipes

Smoked Salmon with Dill and Fennel

Salmon and dill is a combination as old as time. These classic flavors come together in this quick and easy dish. It's a great choice if you are just learning to cook salmon because of its simplicity.

Ingredients (for 4 servings)

- 8 ounces smoked salmon (cut into 4 2-ounce pieces)

- 3 large fennel bulbs (diced)

- 4 tablespoons fresh dill (chopped)

- 2 tablespoons coconut oil

- ¼ teaspoon black pepper

Instructions

Heat a skillet to a medium-high temperature. When warmed, add the coconut oil and tilt to distribute. Add the diced fennel to the pan and saute, until tender. This should take about 10 minutes. Then, add the smoke salmon pieces and heat all the way through. Garnish with fresh dill and black pepper before serving.

Garlic-Ginger Pork Tenders over Cauliflower Rice

Spicy garlic and ginger come together in this dish. You should prepare for it ahead of time, allowing at least 2-3 hours (24 is even better) for the marinade to set into your pork. This recipe requires you to cook the rice in some of the remaining marinade, distributing the flavor through the whole dish.

Ingredients (for 4 servings)

- 1 ½ pound pork tenderloin

- 1 cauliflower head (cut into florets)

- 2 tablespoons fresh ginger (2" of the root, sliced)

- 6 green onions (trimmed and sliced)

- 2 cloves garlic (sliced)

- 1 cup coconut aminos

- 1 cup white wine

- 1 tablespoon coconut oil

- 1 teaspoon salt

Instructions

Prepare the pork tenderloin by cutting it into 1-inch rounds. Put it inside a shallow glass dish or a sealable plastic bag. In a bowl, combine the white wine, coconut aminos, and slices of garlic and ginger. Then, pour the mixed marinade into the dish or bag and turn the meat to distribute. When all the meat is covered, seal it and place it inside the fridge for 2 hours to a full day, flipping the meat or squishing it around several times.

Just before you are ready to cook, bring a large skillet to a medium-high temperature. Remove the tenderloin from the marinade, reserving the remaining marinade for later. Use salt to sprinkle both sides of each tenderloin. When the pan reaches temperature, add coconut oil and tilt to distribute. Once the oil smokes, add the tenderloin and cook for 3-4 minutes per side. The internal temperature should reach 145 degrees.

When the meat is cooked, set it to the side and allow it to rest for 5-10 minutes. While you are waiting, make the cauliflower rice. Pulse the rice in a food processor as you normally would. Remove the ginger slices from the marinade and put the marinade in the pan you used to cook the pork. Once boiling, add the 'rice' and cook to heat through, about 2-3 minutes. Serve by placing the rice and sauce on a plate, topped with the tenderloins and sliced green onions.

Paleo Portobello BLT

This recipe substitutes spinach for lettuce and adds avocado to the mix, but you have traditional BLT flavors. The Portobello makes for a hearty, meaty 'bread' for your sandwich.

Ingredients (for 2 servings)

- 4 medium-sized Portobello mushrooms

- 4 slices bacon (cut in half, cooked through)

- 1 cup spinach

- 1 avocado

- 1 tomato (sliced)

- ¼ yellow onion (sliced)

- ¼ cup cashew butter (or Dijon mustard, depending on your preferred taste)

- 1 tablespoon coconut oil

Instructions

Clean the mushrooms and remove the stem. Use the mustard or cashew butter and spread it on the underside of each cap. Then, layer the cooked bacon and vegetables on two of the caps. Top with the remaining caps.

Preheat the broil. Brush the top of the sandwich with coconut oil and place on a tray. Heat 2-3 minutes in the broiler, until toasty.

Danish Meatloaf

This meatloaf uses eggs and almond flour to hold the meat and vegetable mixture together. The tender loaf is contrasted by crispy bacon cooked on top. Serve alongside your favorite vegetable side.

Ingredients (for 4 servings)

- ½ pound ground turkey

- ½ pound ground pork

- 4 bacon slices

- 6 cremini mushrooms (sliced)

- 1 onion (minced)

- 1 egg (beaten)

- ¼ cup full-fat coconut milk

- 1 tablespoon coconut oil

- 1 teaspoon salt

- ½ teaspoon pepper

Instructions

Set the oven to 400 degrees and allow it to preheat while you prepare the meatloaf. Start by adding the coconut oil to a saute pan and warming to a medium heat. Cook the mushrooms and onions for about 10 minutes, until they become tender and start to brown.

While you are waiting for the mushrooms and onions to cook, mix the turkey and pork with the beaten egg, coconut milk, almond flour, and salt and pepper. Allow the mixture on the stove to cool slightly and add it to the meat mixture, thoroughly mixing it in.

Make a large loaf out of the meat mixture and place in an ungreased baking pan. Layer the bacon across the top of the loaf and cook for 50-60 minutes, until the loaf has cooked all the way through and the bacon is crisp. Either discard the drippings or save them for another recipe.

Sweet and Savory Cacao Nip Pork Chops with Butternut Squash

Pork is a versatile meat, making it the perfect pairing to sweetened butternut squash. The cacao nibs add a savory flavor and a slight crunch to the outside of the tender pork chop.

Ingredients (for 4 servings)

- 4 boneless pork chops (about 4-6 ounces each with fat trimmed off)

- 1 medium-sized butternut squash (skin removed, diced)

- 2 cups spinach

- 1 egg

- 1/3 cup raw cacao nibs (chopped)

- 2 teaspoons + 1 teaspoon coconut oil

- 1 tablespoon raw honey

- ¼ teaspoon cinnamon

- 1 teaspoon salt

- ½ teaspoon pepper

Instructions

Use a meat tenderizer to pound on each side of the chops, to make the meat tenderer. In a small bowl, whisk the egg. Dip each pork chop in this, then season with salt, pepper, and the cacao nibs.

Place a saute pan on the stove on medium heat. Add 2 teaspoons of the coconut oil. When hot, add the squash and cook for about 5 minutes, stirring frequently to prevent sticking. Then, place a second pan on a medium-high temperature and warm the remaining coconut oil. Place the pork chops in this, cooking for 3-4 minutes on each side or until they have reached an internal temperature of 165 degrees.

Once you place the pork inside the pan, add the honey and cinnamon to the butternut squash. Cook an additional 5-6 minutes, seasoning with salt and pepper if you would like. Serve the squash on top of a bed of fresh spinach and serve alongside the spinach.

Springtime Pasta with Shrimp and Asparagus

This fresh, summery-pasta is made with Paleo-friendly zucchini noodles (Zoodles) and offers protein from shrimp. It is a great lunch or can be served alongside dinner.

Ingredients (for 2 servings)

- 4 medium-sized zucchini

- 1 pound asparagus (trimmed and cut into 1-inch slices)

- ½ pound shrimp (deveined, peeled, with tails off)

- ¼ pound cremini mushrooms (sliced)

- 2 gloves garlic (sliced)

- ¼ cup white wine

- 3 tablespoons olive oil

- 2 tablespoons fresh tarragon (finely chopped)

- ¼ teaspoon salt

- ¼ teaspoon pepper

Instructions

Start by creating the zucchini noodles. Trim the zucchini. Then, use a mandolin to create julienne 'noodles' or use a vegetable peeler and peel lengthwise. Place the prepared Zoodles in a strainer. Sprinkle with the salt and toss. Allow the noodles to sit at least 20 minutes, tossing periodically. Then, rinse and remove any excess liquid.

Once drained, add olive oil to a large skillet and allow to warm. Then, add the garlic and mushrooms and saute for 3-5 minutes, until the creminis become soft. Put the asparagus in and toss it with the mushrooms and garlic briefly before adding the white wine. Cover the pan and continue cooking for about 2 minutes, until the asparagus starts to become tender and is bright green in color.

Then, add the fresh tarragon, shrimp, and pepper to the pan. Cook an additional 2-3 minutes, until the shrimp is cooked through and bright pink in color. Once the asparagus mixture is finished, toss with the Zoodles and serve.

Beef and Vegetable Asian-Style Wrap

Instead of a highly-processed tortilla shell, this wrap makes use of a crisp piece of Iceberg or Bibb lettuce. Flavors like fish sauce, coconut aminos, ginger, and select vegetables come together for an Asian experience.

Ingredients (for 2 servings)

For the wraps:

- 1 pound ground beef

- 6 large lettuce leaves (intact)

- ¼ head green cabbage (shredded)

- 4 button mushrooms (sliced)

- 2 cloves garlic (minced)

- 1 onion (chopped)

- 1 tablespoon fresh ginger (chopped)

- 1 tablespoon fish sauce

- 1 tablespoon coconut aminos

- 1 tablespoon apple cider vinegar

For the garnish:

- 2 green onions (chopped)

- 1 carrot (shredded)

- ¼ head green cabbage (shredded)

Instructions

Warm a skillet to medium heat and add the onions and ground beef. Cook about 7-8 minutes, until thoroughly browned. Then, stir in the ginger and garlic, cooking for an additional 1-2 minutes until fragrant.

Next, add the cabbage and mushrooms and cook for 5-6 minutes, until they become soft. Stir in the fish sauce, aminos, and vinegar and cook an additional minute, until heated all the way through.

Set this to the side and assemble the garnish by tossing the ingredients together in a bowl. Spoon the beef mixture into lettuce leaves and top with the vegetables for garnish.

Coconut and Lemongrass Chicken Drumsticks

These tender wings have the fresh flavors of coconut water and lemongrass. They are also made in the crock pot, which means less work for you and low risk of your meat overcooking.

Ingredients

- 10 chicken drumsticks (skin-off)

- 4 cloves garlic (minced)

- 1 cup + ¼ cup coconut milk

- 1 stalk (about 5-inches) lemongrass (trimmed, with the outer skin removed)

- ¼ cup green onions (chopped)

- 3 tablespoons coconut aminos

- 2 tablespoons fish sauce

- 2-3 inches fresh ginger

- 1 onion (thinly sliced)

- 1 teaspoon five spice powder

- 1 teaspoon salt

- ½ teaspoon pepper

Instructions

Add the chicken drumsticks to a Ziploc bag or a large bowl and coat with the salt and pepper. Set to the side. Then, add 1 cup of the coconut milk, coconut aminos, ginger, lemongrass, garlic, and five spice powder to a food processor or blender and pulse until smooth.

Pour the prepared marinade into the bowl with the chicken and toss to coat. In the slow cooker, layer the onions across the bottom. Then, add the chicken and marinade on top. Cook on low heat for 4-5 hours. For a creamy sauce, remove the chicken from the crock pot when done cooking and place the remaining marinade and onions in the blender. Add the additional ¼ cup of coconut milk and blend until combined.

Hearty Turkey Chili

Even though chili is thought of as a cool-weather meal, this hearty chili has summer vegetables. This makes it perfect for cool summer nights.

Ingredients (for 4 servings)

- 1 ½ pounds ground turkey

- 4 bacon slices (diced)

- 1 can (28 ounces) crushed tomatoes (no additives)

- 2 medium-sized zucchini (diced)

- 1 onion (diced)

- 1 jalapeno pepper (seeded and minced)

- 2 cloves garlic (minced)

- 1 yellow bell pepper (diced)

- 2 cups chicken stock

- 2 tablespoons parsley (chopped)

- 1 tablespoon chili powder

- 1 teaspoon oregano

- 1 teaspoon cumin

- ¼ teaspoon salt

- ¼ teaspoon chili powder

- 1/8 teaspoon pepper

Instructions

Add the diced bacon to the bottom of a large pot and cook over medium heat until crisp. Remove the pieces with a slotted spoon and place on paper towels to drain. Then, add zucchini, onions, and peppers to the pot with the bacon grease and cook about 7 minutes, until soft. Add the seasonings and minced garlic and cook an additional minute.

Then, stir in salt and pepper and add the ground turkey. Cook about 10 minutes, until the turkey is browned. Stir as it cooks so all the ingredients are mixed together. Once cooked, add the chicken broth and canned tomatoes. Turn down the heat to a simmer and cook for 30-40 minutes until the chili thickens. Top with the parsley and reserved bacon.

Creamy Broccoli and Chicken Casserole

This casserole is made authentic with crispy almonds and bacon instead of a breadcrumb topping. Its creamy texture is not what you'd expect from a Paleo dish since its void of dairy products, but it is incredibly delicious.

Ingredients (for 4 servings)

- 4-6 ounces of boneless, skinless chicken breasts

- 1 cup full-fat coconut milk

- ½ cup chicken stock

- ¾ cauliflower head (thinly sliced)

- ½ broccoli head (thinly sliced)

- ½ pound white button mushrooms (sliced)

- 4 bacon slices (diced and cooked until crispy)

- ½ cup almonds (sliced)

- 1 egg

- 1 tablespoon coconut oil

- ½ teaspoon salt

- ¼ teaspoon pepper

Instructions

Place a saute pan on the stove and warm to a medium-high temperature. Add the oil once it is warmed. While you are waiting, use salt and pepper to season your chicken. Saute for 7-8 minutes before flipping and cooking the other side until cooked all the way through. When cooked, let the chicken cool until you can handle it and cut into 1-inch pieces.

Set the oven to 350 degrees to preheat. Add the ingredients of the casserole in layers- the broccoli, the mushrooms, the cauliflower, and the chicken.

Use a medium bowl to whisk the chicken broth, coconut milk, and egg together. Once combined, pour this mixture onto the layers and cover with aluminum foil. Place in the oven for 30 minutes. Then, remove the cover and add the almonds and bacon. Bake about 5-10 minutes until the casserole is hot and bubbling and the almonds are lightly toasted. Let the dish sit for at least 10 minutes before cutting, so the liquids set.

Crock Pot Kalua Pig

Traditional Kalua pig takes a whole day to cook over an outdoor smoke pit. Since not all of us have the space (or the time) for this method, this Paleo-friendly Kalua pig recipe has been adapted to the crock pot.

Ingredients (for 10 servings)

- 5 pound Boston pork butt roast (can be bone-in or bone-out)

- 3 bacon slices (thick-cut)

- 5 cloves garlic (peeled)

- 1 ½ tablespoons coarse salt

Instructions

Take the bacon and line the slow cooker with it. Then, place the pork butt on a cutting board and remove the skin if you would like. Salt all the sides of the roast and place it inside the slow cooker on top of the bacon. Roast this for 12-16 hours on the low heat setting. Do not worry about adding any liquid- the roast and bacon fat will make their own.

Once the meat easily falls apart, carefully remove it from the mixture. Shred with 2 forks on a plate or cutting board and place in a large bowl. Test the flavor of the meat. If necessary, add some of the reserved liquid until the Kalua pork is juicy and flavorful.

Roasted Tomatoes Stuffed with Sausage

Sweet, juicy tomatoes are filled with seasoned sausage and roasted in the oven. These are a little small, so 1 ½ tomatoes make up a portion. You can also make them heartier by serving alongside cauliflower rice or another delicious Paleo-side.

Ingredients (for 4 servings)

- 1 pound ground pork sausage (seasoned)

- 6 large tomatoes

- 1 onion (chopped)

- 6 white button mushrooms (sliced)

- 3 tablespoons cilantro (for garnish)

Instructions

Set the oven to 350 degrees to preheat. While you are waiting, place a skillet over medium-high heat and add the sausage, mushrooms, and onions. Cook about 8-10 minutes, until completely browned.

While the sausage is cooking, cut the tops off the tomatoes. Use a spoon to remove the seeds and juices and stir them into the skillet. Place the tomatoes with the bottoms down on a greased baking tray.

Once the sausage is browned, drain the moisture and leftover fat from the pan. Then, spoon it into tomato cups and bake for 10-15 minutes. Garnish with the chopped cilantro before serving.

Crunchy Chicken Fingers

This recipe proves that you don't need grain to enjoy crispy, 'breaded' chicken. Almond flour is baked onto tender chicken in this tasty recipe. You can enjoy these crispy tenders on top of a salad, with a Paleo-friendly dip (you can find some ideas in the next section of the book), or by themselves.

Ingredients (for 4 servings)

- 1 pound skinless, boneless chicken breasts

- 3 egg whites (beaten briefly)

- ¾ cup almond flour

- 1 tablespoon olive oil

- ¼ cup arrowroot powder

- 1 teaspoon salt

- 1 teaspoon cumin

- 1 teaspoon paprika

- ½ teaspoon black pepper

- ½ teaspoon cayenne pepper

- ½ teaspoon garlic powder

Instructions

Start by setting the oven to 375 degrees to preheat. Line a baking sheet with foil and place a wire rack on top. Then, prepare the chicken by cutting it into strips that are 1-2 inches wide. Set these to the side.

Get 3 shallow plates or bowls. In the first, put the arrowroot first. In the second, add the egg whites and whisk them slightly. Add the almond flour and spices in the last bowl and mix to combine. Coat the chicken by covering it in the arrowroot powder and then shaking it off. Then, dip it in the egg whites and dredge it on the flour. Place the chicken directly onto the wire rack and repeat for each individual chicken tender.

When all the chicken is coated, bake it for 20-25 minutes. They should be golden brown, crispy, and cooked all the way through.

Sage-Infused Portobello and Beef Burgers

Flavor is the key component of this savory recipe. Serve alongside your favorite side with some of your favorite burger toppings or place on top of a lettuce wrap with lettuce, onions, Paleo mayonnaise (you can find this recipe in the next section of the book) or whatever other Paleo-friendly ingredients you may enjoy.

Instructions (for 2 servings)

- 1 pound 85/15 lean ground beef

- ¼ pound baby Portobello mushrooms

- 2 tablespoons + 2 tablespoons olive oil

- 3 garlic cloves (minced)

- 2 tablespoons fresh sage (minced)

- 1 teaspoon black pepper

Instructions

Set the oven to preheat to 350 degrees as you clean the mushrooms. Then, cut them into quarters and set on a baking sheet. Bake for 15-20 minutes, until the mushrooms cook down to half their size. While you are waiting, add 2 tablespoons of the olive oil to a skillet over medium heat. Add the sage and garlic and cook for 2-3 minutes.

Add the sage and garlic mixture to a food processor. When they are done, add the roasted mushrooms as well. Process until the mushrooms are coarsely chopped. Add this mixture to a large bowl and combine with the hamburger and black pepper until combined.

245

Warm the skillet you used to fry the garlic and sage to warm the remaining 2 tablespoons of olive oil over medium heat. Cook for about 5 minutes on each side, until cooked all the way through.

Rosemary Grilled Chicken Breast Wrapped with Bacon

The savory flavors of rosemary and garlic are grilled into this chicken breast. It's wrapped with a strip of bacon for added fat. Serve with your favorite Paleo-friendly side.

Ingredients (for 4 servings)

- 1 pound skinless, boneless chicken breasts

- 4 thick bacon slices

- 8 sprigs fresh rosemary

- 4 teaspoons garlic powder

- 1 teaspoon salt

- ½ teaspoon pepper

- Oil for the grill grate

Instructions

Oil the grill grate and set to medium-high heat. Allow it to preheat while you prepare the chicken breasts. Use the garlic, salt, and pepper to season the chicken. Then, place 2 sprigs of rosemary on each breast. Use a slice of bacon to hold the rosemary in place, securing with a toothpick if necessary.

Place the chicken on the grill for 8 minutes before flipping and cooking an additional 8 minutes. Cook until the temperature is 165 degrees internally and there is no pink in the middle.

Creamy Coconut Clam Chowder

This chowder pairs a creamy broth of coconut with protein-rich clams and bacon and filling sweet potatoes. It is hearty enough to be eaten for lunch or dinner.

Ingredients (for 6 servings)

- 1 cup chopped clams (drained, with liquid reserved)

- 2 medium-sized sweet potatoes

- 1 can full-fat coconut milk

- 6 bacon slices

- 2 celery stalks (chopped)

- 2 carrots (sliced)

- ½ onion (diced)

- 2 cloves garlic (minced)

- 2 tablespoons arrowroot powder

- 2 tablespoons olive oil

- 1 tablespoon fresh parsley (chopped)

- ½ teaspoon Italian seasoning

- ½ teaspoon salt

- ½ teaspoon pepper

- ¼ teaspoon cayenne pepper

Instructions

Add the sweet potatoes, celery, and carrots to a large pot and add just enough water to cover them. Cook on medium high heat for about 10 minutes, until tender. Set this to the side, without draining the liquid.

As you are waiting, cook the bacon over medium heat. Remove from the pan and place on top of paper towels or a rack, so the grease drains. Add the onions and garlic to the bacon grease. Cook about 5-7 minutes, until the onions are soft. Then, push this over to one side of the pan and add the clams on the other. Saute for about 4 minutes, being careful not to overcook.

When the clams are cooked, remove them and the onions to the pot with the sweet potatoes and veggies. Then, crumble the bacon into the pot.

Next, use a small pan to heat the arrowroot powder and lard over medium low heat. When well combined, slowly add the coconut milk. Stir the mixture constantly until it thickens, being sure it does not come to a boil. Stir in the seasonings when hot and then add the coconut milk mixture and the clam juice that was reserved to the pot. Heat the pot until the chowder is hot, but be careful that it does not come to a boil or your soup will burn.

Beef and Liver Mediterranean-Style Eggplant

Liver has a distinct taste, making it a food that not everyone enjoys. Still, mixing the liver with beef as you do in this recipe and using Mediterranean flavors allows you to get all the nutrients of liver without the strong taste.

Ingredients (for 4 servings)

- 2 medium-sized eggplants
- ¾ pound ground beef
- ¼ pound veal liver (ground)
- ½ cup walnuts (toasted, chopped)
- 6 tomatoes (diced, with juices retained)
- 1 onion (diced)
- 2 cloves garlic (minced)
- 2 tablespoons fresh mint (chopped)
- 1 tablespoon balsamic vinegar
- 1 teaspoon oregano
- ¼ teaspoon salt
- 1/8 teaspoon pepper

Instructions

Set the oven to 400 degrees to preheat. Cut the eggplants, long ways. Use a sharp knife to score the flesh of the eggplant, being careful not to pierce the skin. Create a crisscross pattern inside the eggplant, with each line about 1" apart from the others going the same direction.

Use the olive oil to coat the flesh of the eggplant. Then, lay with the flesh-side down on a baking sheet and put in the oven for 25-30 minutes, until the eggplant becomes soft and tender.

While you are waiting, add the liver, beef, garlic, and onion to a skillet and brown over medium heat. When cooked all the way through, add the tomatoes and oregano to the mixture. Turn down the temperature to a simmer and stir in the salt and pepper. Cook until the tomatoes start to break down, about 10-15 minutes. Then, stir in the balsamic vinegar.

Once the eggplants are cooked, top with the beef and tomato mixture. Sprinkle the chopped mint and walnuts on top when you are ready to serve.

Cilantro Lime Pork Tacos

Bright flavors come together in this dish. The perfectly seasoned pork and toppings are placed on top of a crisp butter leaf, the perfect substitute for a processed tortilla shell.

Ingredients (for 4 servings)

- 8 large butter leaves (intact)

- 1 pound pork tenderloin (fat trimmed and cut into thin strips, less than 1/2-inch each)

- 2 tomatoes (diced)

- 2 avocadoes (peeled, pitted, and sliced)

- 1 red onion (diced)

- 1 jalapeno pepper (seeded and minced)

- ½ cup chicken broth

- 3 tablespoons fresh cilantro (chopped)

- 3 tablespoons lime juice

- ½ teaspoon salt

- ¼ teaspoon pepper

Instructions

Use the salt and pepper to season the pork strips, tossing them to coat. Then, warm a skillet to medium-high heat and add the coconut oil. Once it starts to smoke, add the pork and cook 4-5 minutes, until lightly browned. Set this aside in a bowl.

Use the same pan to cook the onion and jalapeno. Be cautious of adding jalapeno seeds to the pan, since they will smoke. If you want jalapeno seeds for added heat, stir them in once the jalapeno and onion mixture is tender, about 5-7 minutes.

When the onion is tender, stir in the broth and tomatoes. Allow this to simmer over a low heat for 2-3 minutes, scraping the bottom of the pan to knock the browned bits loose. Then, add the pork and accumulated juices to the pan. Stir in the lime juice and cook 5-10 minutes, until the pork has cooked all the way through.

To serve, place the pork mixture inside the butter leaves. Add avocado slices and chopped cilantro before serving.

Paleo Supreme Pizza

Sausage, vegetables, and Paleo-friendly crust come together in this tasty recipe that will satisfy your pizza craving. Plus, who doesn't love pizza?

Ingredients (for 2 servings)

- 1 cup almond flour

- 1 sausage (cut into ½ inch thick slices)

- 2 eggs (beaten)

- 4 white button mushrooms (sliced)

- 2 cloves garlic (minced)

- 1 red bell pepper (diced)

- ½ cup grape tomatoes (halved)

- ½ cup no-sugar added marinara sauce

- 3 tablespoons almond butter

- 2 teaspoons + 1 teaspoon olive oil

- ½ teaspoon fennel seed

- ½ teaspoon oregano

- ½ teaspoon salt

Instructions

Set the oven to 350 degrees to preheat. Add the almond flour to a bowl with the beaten eggs, almond butter, and salt. Use 2 teaspoons of the olive oil to grease a baking sheet. Spread the pizza 'dough' until you form a ¼"-inch thick crust. Put this in the oven for 10 minutes.

While the crust is cooking, add the rest of the olive oil to a skillet and bring to medium-high heat. Cook the sliced sausage, mushrooms, and onions until the sausage becomes brown and the onions and mushrooms start to become tender. Set this to the side and use the pan to cook the red pepper and garlic for 3-5 minutes, until just tender. Do not overcook any of the vegetables, since they will cook longer in the oven.

When you are ready to remove the crust from the oven, carefully cover it with the marinara sauce. Add the vegetables and sausage to the top and sprinkle with fennel seed and oregano. Return to the oven for about 20 minutes. Then, add the halved tomatoes to the top of the pizza and bake an additional 5-10 minutes. Use caution when lifting this out of the pan, since the crust will not firm up quite as much as traditional pizza dough.

Chapter 4: Paleo Sides, Soups, Dips, Dressings, and Salads

Zucchini Fritters

These tasty bites make a great snack, or a side to a burger or chicken dish. You can alter the recipe by adding ingredients like bacon, green onions, broccoli, or other veggies. Plain yogurt and homemade guacamole (or mashed avocado) taste great as a dip or a topping.

Ingredients (for 2 servings)

- 3 eggs

- 2 medium-sized zucchini

- 2 tablespoons bacon grease (or coconut oil)

- 1 tablespoon coconut flour

- 1 teaspoon salt

- ¼ teaspoon black pepper

Instructions

Prepare the zucchini by hand-shredding it or roughly chopping it in a food processor, depending on how you want the consistency of your fritters. Set to the side on a plate, blotting with a paper towel if the zucchini is especially wet.

Crack the eggs into a large bowl and whisk together. Then, sift the coconut flour in and mix together. Add the shredded zucchini, salt, and pepper to the bowl and mix to combine.

Set the fritter mix to the side while you warm a cast iron skillet over a medium-low temperature. Add the grease (or oil) once the skillet has warmed. Then, create fritters and fry them in the grease, a few minutes per side until browned and cooked all the way through.

Avocado-Cilantro Dressing/Dip

This recipe makes a great dip or dressing. It is packed full of healthy fats from the avocado and flavor from lime and cilantro.

Ingredients (for 8 servings)

- ¾ packed cup fresh cilantro (chopped)

- 2 green onions (chopped)

- ½ avocado (skinned and pitted)

- 1 clove garlic

- 1/3 cup avocado oil

- ¼ cup lime juice

- ¼ cup full-fat coconut milk

- 1 teaspoon salt

- ½ teaspoon pepper

Instructions

Add all the ingredients to a blender and mix until all the ingredients are smooth and combined. If the consistency is too thick for your preference, add additional olive oil or coconut milk. You can store leftovers for about 4 days, but you will need to blend before serving since the ingredients will separate.

Sautéed Sweet Potatoes

Sweet potatoes are one of the high-carb foods that you can eat without feeling guilty on the Paleolithic Diet. This is a hash-brown style dish that goes great alongside eggs for breakfast or a meat for lunch or dinner.

Ingredients (for 2 servings)

- 1 large sweet potato (grated)

- 1 tablespoon coconut oil

- ¼ teaspoon cinnamon

- 1/8 teaspoon nutmeg

Instructions

Place a skillet on a stove to a medium temperature. Once warm, add the coconut oil. Tilt the pan slightly to disperse and add the grated sweet potatoes. Sprinkle the cinnamon and nutmeg on top and stir to combine. Then, saute on either side until tender, cooking longer if you want them to be browned like traditional hash browns.

Basic Salad Dressing

This recipe provides a base that you can add different herbs to as you learn what you like on different Paleo salads. Some good options include chives, tarragon, rosemary, thyme, basil, oregano, and chives. Since you can easily adjust the recipe for the flavors you want, choose any combination of herbs and create something that tastes great to your palate.

Ingredients (for 8 servings)

- 1 cup extra virgin olive oil

- 1 clove garlic (minced)

- ¼ cup balsamic vinegar

- 1 tablespoon lemon juice

- 1 teaspoon herb or herbs of your choice (adjust as needed)

- 1 teaspoon raw honey

- 1 teaspoon Dijon mustard

- 1 teaspoon salt

- ½ teaspoon pepper

Instructions

Add the balsamic vinegar, minced garlic, lemon juice, honey, and mustard to a medium bowl and mix together until they are all well incorporated. Alternatively, you could use a blender. Once they are mixed, slowly add the olive oil as you continue to whisk or blend.

Next, taste the dressing. Add the salt and pepper, as well as the herbs. Adjust until you reach your desired taste. This dressing can be stored in an airtight container for as long as a week.

Apple Coleslaw

Tangy Granny Smith apples, crisp cabbage, and sweet bell peppers come together in this recipe. This is coated with a sweet and tangy dressing.

Ingredients

- ¼ cup olive oil

- 1 Granny Smith apple (peeled, cored, and grated)

- ½ cabbage head (chopped)

- Juice of 1 lemon

- 1 red bell pepper (chopped)

- 1 celery stalk (chopped)

- 2 tablespoons raw, organic honey

- 1 ½ teaspoons celery seed

- ½ teaspoon salt

Instructions

Add the prepared apples, cabbage, bell pepper, and celery to a large bowl and toss to combine. In a separate bowl, whisk together the remaining ingredients. Pour this over the fruits and vegetables and stir gently to combine.

Creamy Garlic-Pepper Dip

This creamy dip recipe tastes great as a spread for Paleo bread, a dip for veggies or chicken tenders, on sandwiches, and more. You can alter the flavor with different herbs if you choose.

Ingredients (for 4 servings)

- 1 cup raw cashews

- ½ cup olive oil

- 2 cloves garlic

- 2 tablespoon nutritional yeast

- 2 tablespoons lemon juice

- 1 teaspoon pepper

- ½ teaspoon salt

Instructions

Add the cashews to shallow dish. Add cold water until it just covers them and soak for 3-4 hours. Be careful of over-soaking, because this will alter the flavor of the cashews.

Once you are ready, drain the water from the cashews and add them to the blender with the other ingredients. Process until completely smooth. If it seems to thick, you may need to add a little water to the blender. Adjust the seasoning as needed and blend again. Then, store in an airtight container for up to 3 days in the refrigerator.

Shrimp Cakes

Healthy fats and nutrients from assorted vegetables come together in these delicious cakes. They can be served as a side or even an easy meal.

Ingredients (for 4 servings)

- 1 pound shrimp (de-veined, peeled, with tails off)

- ½ cup almond flour

- ½ cup fresh cilantro (chopped)

- 1 egg

- 2 green onions (thinly sliced)

- 1 red bell pepper (diced)

- 2 garlic cloves (minced)

- 3 tablespoons coconut oil

- 1 tablespoon raw honey

- 1 tablespoon lime juice

- ½ teaspoon sea salt

- ¼ teaspoon ground chipotle

Instructions

Process the shrimp in a food processor until it is finely chopped. Add this to a large bowl with the green onions, pepper, egg, honey, lime juice, cilantro, garlic, and chipotle. Mix well and then create patties that are ½-inch thick. If your mixture is not thick enough, you can add a little almond flour to the mixture.

Once the patties are formed, warm a large skillet and add the coconut oil. When it reaches a medium temperature, add the patties and cook for about 5 minutes on each side until brown in color. Place on a plate lined with paper towels and cook the remaining patties.

Paleo Langostino Lobster Squat Soup

This is a spin on a traditional Mexican soup with tender Langostino lobster pieces, vegetables, and a spicy, savory broth. If you cannot find lobster, this recipe tastes equally delicious when made using shrimp. Either way, it contains plenty of protein and healthy fats.

Ingredients (for 4 servings)

- 2 pounds shelled Langostino lobsters
- 2 cans (6.5 ounces each) chopped clams
- 2 cups water
- 1 cup chicken broth
- 1 can (14.5 ounces) crushed tomatoes (no sugar added)
- 2 carrots (peeled and diced)
- 2 garlic cloves
- 1 onion (chopped)
- 2 large-sized mild-flavored dried chilies (like Guajillo or Anaheim chilies)
- 1 bay leaf
- 1 teaspoon dried oregano
- 1 teaspoon olive oil
- 4 teaspoons cilantro (chopped, for garnish)
- 1 lime (quartered, for garnish)
- 1 teaspoon salt
- ½ teaspoon pepper

Instructions

Add the dried chilies to a bowl and add just enough water to cover them. Soak for 30 minutes. Then, remove from the water, remove the stems, and take out the seeds. Add the chilies to a food processor with the canned tomatoes, garlic, onion, and oregano and blend until pureed.

Next, add the olive oil to a pot and warm over medium-low heat. After it has warmed, add the puree and cook at a simmer for 6 minutes, until fragrant. Next, add the juice from the cans of clams, water, chicken broth, and the bay leaf. Continue to simmer for an additional 5 minutes so the flavors can muddle together.

While the soup base is simmering, prepare the carrots and rinse the Langostinos. Add the carrots and simmer an additional 5 minutes. Then, add the clams and lobsters. Once the pan returns to a simmer, cover with a lid, turn off the heat, and let it sit for 10 minutes. This slow-cooking will flavor the sea food without turning it rubbery and overcooking it.

Taste the soup once 10 minutes has lapsed and add the salt and pepper, using the recommended amounts or adjusting as needed. Additionally, you could add hot sauce or dried red chili flakes if you want additional spice. Before serving, top with the chopped cilantro and 1 of the lime wedges.

Creamy Mushroom Soup

You would think any 'cream' of soup would be off limits, since they involve dairy. This recipe uses avocado to make it creamy, as well as to add healthy fats. The mushrooms and other vegetables also give it plenty of vitamins and nutrients.

Ingredients (for 2 servings)

- 6 white button mushrooms (sliced)

- 2 medium avocados (peeled, with pit removed)

- 1 red bell pepper (diced)

- 2 tomatoes (diced)

- ¼ onion (minced)

- 2 cloves garlic

- Juice of ½ medium-sized grapefruit

- 1 cup water

- 1 cup chicken stock

- 4 tablespoons fresh basil

- 1 tablespoon coconut oil

Instructions

Place the water and chicken stock on the stove and bring to a boil. When hot, add to a food processor with the avocado, garlic cloves, and grapefruit juice. Pulse until it is a smooth consistency and set to the side.

Place a medium pot on the stove and warm to medium-high heat. When warmed, add the coconut oil. Then, put the remaining ingredients in the pan and saute until softened, about 8-10 minutes. Add the mixture from the food processor and cook until hot.

Garlic-Ginger Almond Dressing

This dip/dressing pairs well with chicken, seafood, and other meats. It has Asian-inspired flavors and offers the perfect blend of spicy and sweet. You should note that because of the sesame oil, this is best served without heating.

Ingredients (for 6 servings)

- 5 tablespoons coconut aminos

- 1 green onion (minced)

- ¼ cup sesame oil

- 2 tablespoons almond butter

- 2 cloves garlic

- 1 tablespoon raw honey

- 1 tablespoon fresh ginger (minced)

Instructions

Add all the ingredients to the blender until thoroughly mixed. Always blend just before using, since the oil will cause all the ingredients to separate. This tastes great on vegetables, meat, or salad.

Sweet Potato Fries

These sweet, salty, and crisp fries are the perfect pairing for grilled chicken, a hamburger, or even on top of a steak salad.

Ingredients (for 4 servings)

- 4 medium-sized sweet potatoes

- 3 ½ tablespoons olive oil

- ½ teaspoon salt

- ½ teaspoon cumin

- ¼ teaspoon black pepper

Instructions

Set the oven to 400 degrees to preheat. Lay a sheet of parchment paper on a baking tray. Cut the potatoes into fries, with or without skin, about ¼-inch thick.

Add the cut sweet potatoes to a large bowl with the olive oil and seasoning. Toss to coat and place in a single layer on the baking tray. Do not overcrowd, because this will make your fries soggy. Bake for 15 minutes and flip before baking an additional 15 minutes. The sweet potato fries should be lightly browned and crisp.

Roasted Roots Ratatouille

Root vegetables are at the heart of this savory dish, with pine nuts for crunch and a little added protein. This makes a great snack or a side to a meat of your choosing.

Ingredients (for 4 servings)

- 1 eggplant (diced)

- 2 sweet potatoes (peeled and diced)

- ½ butternut squash (peeled and cubed)

- 2 carrots (diced)

- 1 zucchini (diced)

- 1 red onion (chopped)

- ¼ cup toasted pine nuts

- ¼ cup fresh parsley (chopped)

- 2 tablespoons olive oil

- 1 teaspoon fresh thyme

- ¼ teaspoon salt

- 1/8 teaspoon pepper

Instructions

Set the oven to 400 degrees so it can preheat. Then, prepare a baking tray by lining it with a sheet of parchment paper. Add the carrots, butternut squash, and sweet potatoes to the tray and toss with olive oil and the herbs. Then, cook in the oven for 15 minutes.

Carefully add the remaining vegetables to the tray and stir.
Return to the oven to roast until the vegetables have browned
lightly and become tender. This should take 20-25 minutes.
Just before serving, mix the roasted vegetables with the pine
nuts.

Italian-Style Garlic and Herb Spaghetti Squash

Plump tomatoes, slices of garlic, and select herbs give an authentic Italian taste to this side. It pairs especially well with a main dish of chicken or shrimp.

Ingredients (for 4 servings)

- 2 pounds spaghetti squash (about 1 medium squash)

- 1 cup grape tomatoes (sliced)

- 2 cloves garlic (thinly sliced)

- 2 tablespoons olive oil

- 1 tablespoon fresh basil (chopped, for garnish)

- 1 teaspoon parsley

- 1 teaspoon salt

- ½ teaspoon black pepper

Instructions

Start by setting the oven to 375 degrees to preheat. While you are waiting, prepare the spaghetti squash by cutting it in half. Use a spoon to remove the seeds and place the squash in a baking dish, with the cut side down. Add water until it is about 1/2 an inch high. Cook in the oven for 35-40 minutes, until the squash becomes tender.

Once the squash is cooked, allow it to cool. When you can handle it, use a fork to scrape the squash flesh out, trying not to squish the strands of squash. Set these on a plate, off to the side.

Then, warm the olive oil to medium heat in a large skillet. Add the garlic and cook for 1-2 minutes, being careful not to brown it. Then, add the halved tomatoes and parsley to the pan and cook another 2 minutes, until the tomatoes are soft and warm. Remove the pan from the heat and add the spaghetti squash, tossing to combine. Top with fresh basil before serving.

Simple Cauliflower Rice

For many people, rice is a difficult staple to give up when they go Paleo. With its flexible flavor and ability to be textured like rice, however, it is not packed full of carbohydrates.

Ingredients (for 4 servings)

- 1 cauliflower head (with most of the stem removed, cut into florets)

- 2 tablespoons coconut oil

- 1 tablespoon salt

- 1 teaspoon pepper

- Seasonings of your choice (depending on the recipe, you could use ginger, garlic, curry, lime juice, cilantro, or any other seasoning)

Instructions

Add the cauliflower florets to a food processor and pulse until it has a coarse consistency, similar to rice. Do not over-process. Season with salt, pepper, and your choice of seasonings and pulse once more to combine.

Then, place a large skillet on the stove and bring it to a medium-high temperature. Add the coconut oil and tilt to distribute. Then, add the cauliflower and saute for 4-5 minutes, until the cauliflower is tender and warmed all the way through.

Paleo Mayonnaise

Mayonnaise is the perfect complement to a sandwich. Unfortunately, it is not usually Paleo friendly. This easy-to-make version always thickens and can be stored for up to a week in the fridge in an airtight container.

Ingredients (for 8 servings)

- 2 large, pastured egg yolks

- ½ cup avocado oil

- ½ cup extra virgin olive oil

- Juice of ½ lemon

- 1 teaspoon Dijon mustard

- ¼ teaspoon salt

Instructions

Add the avocado and olive oils together in a bowl and set to the side. In a separate bowl, add the lemon juice to the egg yolks. Use a hand mixer or quickly beat the ingredients to blend. Slowly add in the oils, continuing to blend a small drizzle. You will need to beat for at least 4-5 minutes for the oil to be completely incorporated. When you have a thick mixture, blend in the mustard and salt until well incorporated.

Paleo Egg Drop Soup

Chinese food is probably one of the biggest no-nos on the Paleo Diet, especially since it usually contains high levels of MSGs and other processed ingredients. This doesn't mean that you can't enjoy it with the right substitutions though and this egg drop soup is proof of that.

Ingredients (for 2 servings)

- 3 cups chicken stock
- 2 eggs
- 2 teaspoons fish sauce
- 1 teaspoon hot chili peppers (thinly sliced, for garnish)
- 2 teaspoons fresh cilantro (chopped, for garnish)
- 2 scallions (thinly sliced, for garnish)
- ½ teaspoon salt

Instructions

Add the stock to a medium sauce pan and warm to a medium-high heat. Add the fish sauce and salt, adjusting as needed. Once it has reached a rolling boil, it is time to add the eggs.

Place the eggs in a small bowl and whisk together until well-combined. If you would like, you can add more salt and fish sauce to the eggs to taste. Once the eggs are ready, remove the soup pot from the heat. Slowly whisk in the eggs- they should cook as they come into contact with the broth, making thin and wispy egg strands rather than chunks. Top with the chili peppers, scallions, and cilantro and enjoy.

French Dressing

This sweet and savory dressing is the perfect complement to a salad, which is great since most retail dips are not approved for the Paleo Diet.

Ingredients (for 6 servings)

- 1 can (6 ounces) tomato paste (minimally processed)

- 3 tablespoons Paleo mayonnaise (recipe can be found on the previous page)

- ½ cup olive oil

- ¼ cup raw honey

- ¼ cup champagne vinegar

- ¼ onion (chopped)

- 1 clove garlic

- 1 teaspoon paprika

- 1 teaspoon Worcestershire sauce

- ¼ teaspoon salt

- ¼ teaspoon pepper

Instructions

Add all the ingredients except the olive oil to a blender. Process until it has a smooth consistency. Then, slowly add the olive oil and blend an additional 2-3 minutes, until completely incorporated. This stores for as long as week.

Paleo Bread

This recipe has a hearty, grainy flavor like most breads, but it is grain-free and Paleo-friendly. You can enjoy it toasted for breakfast or use it to make a tasty sandwich.

Ingredients (for 10 servings)

- 3 cups almond flour

- 7 eggs

- 6 tablespoons flax seeds (ground)

- 3 tablespoons coconut flour

- 1 ½ tablespoons raw honey

- 1 ½ tablespoons coconut oil (melted, plus more for coating the pan)

- 1 ½ tablespoons apple cider vinegar

- 1 ½ teaspoons baking soda

- ½ teaspoon salt

Instructions

Start by setting the oven to 350 degrees to preheat. Use a stand mixer (or a food processor) to combine the ground flax, two types of flour, baking soda, and salt. Pulse until well combined. Then, mix in the eggs and mix until combined. Finally, add in the remaining ingredients.

When well mixed, prepare a bread pan by greasing it with coconut oil. Use a spatula to help you scrape all the batter into the pan. Bake for 30-40 minutes, until the bread is cooked all the way through and you can insert a knife into the center and have it come out clean. If the top browns too much, you can put a sheet of foil over it while it finishes cooking. Let the bread cool completely before slicing it.

Broccoli Soup

This nutrient- and vitamin-packed soup has rich broccoli flavor that is enhanced with chicken broth, lemon, and bacon. Even without the cheese that is usually found in this type of soup, it is hot, creamy, and delicious.

Ingredients (for 4 servings)

- 3 broccoli heads

- 5 cups chicken stock

- 2 small turnips (quartered)

- Juice of 1 medium lemon

- ¾ cup unsweetened almond milk

- 1/3 cup full-fat coconut cream

- 8 bacon slices (cooked and crumbled)

- 1 onion (chopped)

- 2 tablespoons coconut oil

- ¼ teaspoon salt

- 1/8 teaspoon pepper

Instructions

Place a large soup pan on the stove and warm the chicken stock. As its warming, heat a skillet to medium heat and melt the coconut oil. Add the turnips, onions, lemon juice, and salt and pepper to the skillet and cook for 5 minutes, until the vegetables are slightly softened.

Then, stir the broccoli into the skillet and continue cooking for 5 minutes. Turn down the heat to a simmer and stir in the chicken broth. Cover this and simmer for 10-15 minutes, until the broccoli becomes tender. Then, add the heated mixture to a blender and process until it has a smooth consistency. Mix in the almond milk and coconut cream before returning to the stove, in the pot you used to heat the chicken stock. Heat over medium-low until hot all the way through and top with bacon crumbles.

Chapter 5: Paleo Snacks and Desserts

Bacon Wrapped Dates

This recipe is baked, bringing out the sweet dates to contrast beautifully with the crispy, salty bacon. Four of these bites makes a filling snack! To keep the bites from unraveling while they cook, pierce them with toothpicks before putting them in the oven.

Ingredients (for 4 servings)

- 16 Medjool dates

- 8 slices bacon (halved)

- 16 whole almonds

Instructions

Set the oven to 375 degrees to preheat. Then, use a knife to slightly open a date. Press an almond inside each. Then, wrap half a strip of bacon around the date. As you wrap these, place on a baking tray with the seam of the bacon facing down. Cook for 7 minutes. Then, flip and cook an additional 7-10 minutes, until the bacon becomes crispy. These bites taste great warm or cold.

Coconut Cashew Cream and Banana Tart

The sweet, tropical flavors of this dish come together on top of a Paleo-friendly crust. Delicious cashew cream and coconut fill this pie and bananas are assembled on top.

Ingredients (for 10 servings)

- 1 ½ cups dates (pitted)

- 1 ½ cups pecans

- 1 cup cashews (soaked and drained)

- 4 bananas (firm, but ripe)

- ¾ cup unsweetened coconut (shredded)

- ½ cup water

- 1 vanilla bean (split open and scraped)

- 2 tablespoons + 2 teaspoons maple syrup (plus more to taste, if needed)

Instructions

Add the pecans and the salt to a food processor and pulse until coarsely chopped. Then, add the dates and pulse about 15-20 seconds, just until well combined. Finally, add the syrup to the blender and pulse until combined. The mixture should stick to itself slightly. This will be the crust of the pie- press it into a 9-inch pie plate and set to the side.

Next, make the filling. Grind the cashews in the blender until they have a coarse consistency. Add the vanilla scrapings, water, and syrup to the cashew mixture and blend until smooth. You want the filling to have a consistency similar to very thick pancake batter. Remove 2 tablespoons of coconut for the garnish and put the remainder in the blender, mixing until just combined. Use this to create an even layer in the prepared piecrust.

Slice the bananas, using a slightly diagonal angle. Use the banana 'coins' to create round rows, starting at the crust and slightly overlapping as you move inward. Top with the remaining coconut and serve.

Guacamole Deviled Eggs

Rich avocado and cooked egg yolks in this spin on a traditional deviled egg. This meal is packed full of healthy fats from the avocados and protein from the eggs for a filling snack or side.

Ingredients (for 2 servings)

- 1 large avocado

- 4 eggs (hard-boiled)

- 1 teaspoon lemon juice

- ½ teaspoon hot pepper sauce (or to taste)

- 1 ½ teaspoons red pepper flakes (or to taste)

- 1/2 teaspoon salt

- ¼ teaspoon black pepper

Instructions

Slice the avocado in half and pit it, before removing the flesh to a food processor. Slice the eggs the long way, removing the yolk and adding it to the food processor with the avocado.

Set the egg whites to the side and add the hot sauce, pepper flakes, lemon juice, salt, and pepper to the processor. Then, pulse the ingredients until combined and your desired consistency. You can puree until smooth or leave chunky. Use a spoon to fill the egg whites with the guacamole mixture and enjoy.

Spiced Pumpkin Seeds

This recipe offers traditional fall flavors with something that is always around in the fall- pumpkins! This is a great snack to munch on regardless of where you are. The ingredients for this list are non-specific, since you can use the basic recipe to create small or large batches. You can also change the spices and herbs used to change the flavor.

Ingredients (for 10 servings)

- Raw pumpkin seeds from 1 pumpkin

- 1 tablespoon allspice

- 1 tablespoon cumin

- 1 tablespoon coriander

- 2 tablespoons olive oil

- ½ teaspoon salt

- ½ teaspoon pepper

Instructions

Set the oven to 350 degrees to preheat. Boil water in a large or medium pot, depending on the size of your batch, with 1-2 teaspoons of salt to the water. Take the innards of a gutted pumpkin and remove the seeds, cleaning off the bits of pumpkin as you go. Place them inside a strainer and rinse using cold water, until there are no stringy bits or pumpkin meat left on them. They should be white in color.

Once the water has reached a boil, add the seeds and cook for 10 minutes. Strain them through the strainer and rinse. Then, pat the seeds dry using a towel. Add the dried seeds to a large bowl and add 1-2 teaspoons of olive oil. You want them evenly coated, but just barely. Add the spices and toss all the ingredients together.

You may need to do more than one batch of pumpkin seeds, depending on how many you are making. Lay the seeds in a single layer on a baking tray, overlapping them as little as possible. Roast in the oven for 10 minutes and stir. Then, bake the seeds 5-10 minutes longer, carefully removing a few of the seeds and cracking them open to be sure the insides aren't burning (they will be brown if they are). You will know the seeds are done when the outsides are lightly browned and easy to bite through.

Dehydrated Apple Chips

These apple snacks have a crunch. After being slow cooked in the oven, they are dried out. Cinnamon and fresh-squeezed apple juice give this recipe flavor, but you can easily make them with another juice or with other seasonings.

Ingredients (for 4 servings)

- Juice of 5-6 large apples (about 2 cups)

- 2 large apples

- 1 cinnamon stick

- 1 teaspoon cinnamon

Instructions

Set the oven to 250 degrees to preheat. Add the apple juice and cinnamon stick to a large pot and allow it to come to a low boil. Core the 2 apples and remove the tops and bottoms. Cut into slices that are about 1/8-inch thick.

Then, drop the slices into the boiling juice. Cook until the apple slices look translucent, about 4-5 minutes. Take a slotted spoon and carefully remove the slices from the juice. Place on a cloth towel and gently pat dry.

Then, place the chips on a wire cooling rack over a baking tray. The tray will catch excess drips. Bake 30-40 minutes in the oven, until the apples are almost dry when touched and golden brown in color.

Chocolate-Coconut No-Bakes

These no-bake cookies will remind you of a Mounds bar, but without the processed ingredients. You can make the cookies as large or as small as you like, just remember that ¼ of the recipe is a serving.

Ingredients (for 4 servings)

- 1 cup unsweetened coconut flakes

- ½ cup dark chocolate chips (at least 85% dark)

- ¼ cup almond butter

- ¼ cup unsweetened cocoa powder

- 3 tablespoons coconut oil

- 2 tablespoons raw honey

Instructions

Add the chocolate chips and coconut oil to a microwave safe bowl and cook 30 seconds at a time, stirring after each interval until thoroughly melted. Then, stir in the honey, almond butter, and cocoa powder until smooth. Once smooth, stir in the coconut flakes.

Set the mixture to the side while you prepare a baking sheet by covering it with parchment paper. Drop the prepared mixture onto the sheet, using a tablespoon or ice cream scoop. Refrigerate the cookies until they harden.

Cucumber Salmon Bites with Cashew Cheese

Crisp cucumber, smoked salmon, and creamy cashew cheese come together in this recipe. These delicious bites are a great snack, especially since they are best eaten cold.

Ingredients (for 4 servings)

For the bites:

- 1 pound smoked salmon

- 1 medium cucumber

- 2 tablespoons fresh chives

- Cashew cheese

For the cashew cheese:

- 1 ½ cups raw cashews

- ¼ cup water

- Juice of 1 lemon

- 1 clove garlic

- ¼ teaspoon salt

Instructions

Make the cashew cheese first. Set the cashews in a bowl and cover them with the water, using more if needed. Let them sit for 3-4 hours. Then, drain them and put the cashews in a food processor.

Add the remaining ingredients for the cashew cheese to the blender and process until it has a smooth and creamy texture.

You can add a little water if needed to thin the cheese, depending on your desired consistency.

Slice the cucumber into 1/4-inch thick rounds. Add some of the cashew cheese and a tablespoon of salmon to each bite. Place these on a tray and sprinkle with the chives when you are finished.

Easy Watermelon Freeze

This sweet and cool treat is perfect for a summer day. The addition of mint makes this recipe even fresher and provides the watermelon with a contrasting flavor.

Ingredients *(for 2 servings)*

- 4 cups unseeded watermelon (cubed)

- 1 cup water

- Juice of 1 lemon

- ½ medium cantaloupe (cubed)

- 3 tablespoons fresh mint

Instructions

Add the cantaloupe and watermelon to a food processor and blend until smooth. Then, put the mixture into a saucepan over medium heat until it simmers for about 15 minutes.

When the watermelon mixture is almost done, place the mint into another saucepan and cover with the water. Bring to a boil and steep for 3 minutes. Then, strain out the mint leaves and add the water to the melon mixture. Remove the mixture from heat and stir in the lemon juice.

The mixture is now ready to freeze. You can use paper cups, an ice cube tray, or popsicle molds. If you are using a cup or a tray, let the mixture firm up for about an hour before inserting the popsicle stick. Freeze completely, about 4 hours before serving.

Sweet Potato Brownies and Chocolate Icing

This is definitely not a dessert you'd expect to be eating on the Paleo Diet. It is rich in chocolatey flavor. While the sweet potatoes give the brownies their moist texture, you cannot taste them at all in this recipe.

Ingredients (for 12 servings)

For the brownie:

- 1 large sweet potato (baked and peeled)

- 1 cup unsweetened cocoa powder

- 2 tablespoons coconut flour

- 2 eggs

- ½ cup coconut oil (melted)

- ½ cup raw honey

- 1 tablespoon baking powder

- 1 tablespoon vanilla extract

- ½ teaspoon baking soda

For the icing:

- 1 cup dark chocolate chips

- 1/3 cup coconut oil

- 1 tablespoon vanilla extract

Instructions

Set the oven to 365 degrees to preheat. Mash the sweet potatoes and add them to a large bowl with the coconut oil, eggs, honey, and vanilla. Mix to combine. In a separate bowl, add the coconut flour, cocoa powder, baking soda, and baking powder and combine. Stir the dry ingredients into the bowl with the sweet potato mixture.

Set the bowl to the side while you lay parchment paper inside an 8x8 pan. Spread the batter evenly across the bottom and place in the oven for 25-30 minutes. It is done once a toothpick can be inserted and comes out clean. Do not overbake or your brownies will not be as moist.

Once you put the brownies in the oven, start preparing the frosting. Add the coconut oil and chocolate chips together in a pan on the stove. Mix together over low heat until melted and then stir in the vanilla. Remove the pan from the stove and transfer the frosting to the refrigerator. It will need to cool completely before the next step.

Take the frosting and use a hand mixer to whip it until it becomes fluffy. When the brownies are done, allow them to cool before topping with the icing and servings.

Paleo Trail Mix

Trail mix is a great snack, since it requires no preparation, does not need to be refrigerated, and can be enjoyed anywhere. You can use this recipe or alter it slightly to meet your own taste preferences.

Ingredients (for 12 servings)

- 2 cups raw pumpkin seeds (unsalted)

- 2 cups sunflower seed kernels (roasted, unsalted)

- 1 cup almond slivers (roasted, unsalted)

- ¾ cup dried coconut flakes (toasted)

- ¾ cup dried pineapple (diced)

Instructions

Add all the ingredients to a large bowl and toss to combine. Store in an airtight container and enjoy!

'Ice Cream' Bites

These chocolate-covered 'ice cream' bites are sure to satisfy your cravings. The best part about it is they are Paleo-friendly so you don't have to feel guilty about eating a few.

Ingredients (for 6 servings)

- 3 medium-sized bananas (cut into 1-inch pieces and frozen beforehand)
- 7 ounces 80% or higher dark chocolate (finely chopped)
- ¼ cup coconut oil
- 3 tablespoons almonds (toasted and chopped)
- 1 teaspoon vanilla extract
- 1/8 teaspoon salt

Instructions

Add the frozen banana pieces and vanilla extract to a food processor and combine until the mixture is smooth and creamy. Then, place the ice cream in a sealed, airtight container and freeze for 2-3 hours, until it solidifies.

Use a teaspoon or small ice cream scoop to make the balls. You want to have about 24 to eat 4 of the ice cream bites for a serving. Line a baking tray with parchment paper and place the balls on this. Once you are out of ice cream mixture, return to the freezer so they don't melt while you prepare the chocolate.

Add the coconut oil and chocolate shavings and cook in a double boiler until melted. Alternatively, you could microwave for 20-30 seconds at a time until smooth. Use a skewer or fork to pick up each ball and dip it into the chocolate mixture. Top with a few toasted almond pieces and return to the tray. Allow to set for 10-15 minutes in the freezer (or until solid) before eating.

Bacon-Tomato Sweet Potato Bites

Crispy and salty bacon comes together with juicy tomatoes and soft sweet potato for a medley of flavors. They taste good warm or cold, so make some ahead and keep them in the refrigerator for whenever you are hungry.

Ingredients (for 6 servings)

- 2 medium-sized sweet potatoes

- 2 cups grape tomatoes (quartered)

- 6 bacon slices (chopped and crisped in a skillet)

- ¼ cup fresh parsley (chopped)

- 2 tablespoons olive oil

- ¼ teaspoon salt

- 1/8 teaspoon pepper

Instructions

Warm the broiler to the high heat setting and lay a piece of parchment paper on a baking sheet. Slice the sweet potatoes into slices that are 1/8-inch thick. Use half the olive oil to coat the top of the sweet potatoes and sprinkle with the salt. Put these in the broiler until they are slightly charred on top and softened.

While you are waiting, add the remaining olive oil to the crisped bacon, tomatoes, and parsley and toss. Spoon this on the sweet potato slices and season with pepper before serving.

Strawberry Rhubarb Crisp

This sweet and tangy dessert resembles all the flavor of a strawberry-rhubarb pie, but it is free of processed sugar. Instead, natural honey and date sugar are used as sweeteners and the crumble is a gluten-free version.

Ingredients *(for 4 servings)*

- 2 cups fresh strawberries (cleaned and sliced)
- ½ pound rhubarb (peeled and diced)
- ¾ cup almonds (finely diced or coarsely ground)
- ¾ cup coconut oil
- ½ cup unsweetened applesauce
- ½ cup coconut sugar
- ½ cup starch or tapioca flour
- ¼ cup raw honey
- ¼ cup date sugar
- 1/8 cup coconut flour

Instructions

Set the oven to 400 degrees so it can preheat. Add the strawberries and rhubarb to a large bowl with the raw honey, date sugar, and almond flour. Stir to combine. Use oil to coat a 9x9 baking dish and spread the prepared mixture inside. Set this to the side.

Use a medium mixing bowl to combine the 2 flours with coconut sugar, diced almonds, coconut sugar, applesauce, and coconut oil. Stir all the ingredients are distributed throughout.

300

Bake for 35-40 minutes, until the strawberries and rhubarbs have softened and the top has started to brown.

If you choose, you can top with coconut whipped cream. (You can find this recipe next). You can also garnish with fresh slices of rhubarb or strawberries.

Coconut Whipped Cream

Since traditional whipped cream is full of dairy and sugar, you would assume it's something you have to give up on the Paleo Diet. As you choose your coconut milk, be sure it is full-fat. You want to be able to separate the fatty oils of the coconut from the liquid.

Ingredients (for 4 servings)

- 1 can full-fat coconut milk (chilled in the fridge overnight, upside down)

- 1/8 teaspoon cinnamon or nutmeg (optional)

- 1/8 teaspoon vanilla extract (optional)

Instructions

If you turned the can upside down to refrigerate the coconut milk, then it should be separated with the oils on top. Remove the oils and reserve the remaining liquid for another recipe or discard. Add the solidified oil to a medium bowl and use a wire whisk or electric beater to beat it until it starts to form soft peaks. Add in the vanilla and cinnamon if you are using them and continue to beat until the coconut cream reaches your desired consistency.

Almond Macaroons

This delicious, buttery recipe melts in your mouth. It offers plenty of almond taste and satisfaction for your sweet tooth with a Paleo-friendly recipe.

Ingredients (for 6 servings)

- 1 ¼ cups almonds

- 2 egg whites (beaten)

- ¼ cup raw honey

- 1 teaspoon lemon juice

- 1 teaspoon lemon zest

- 1/8 teaspoon cinnamon

Instructions

Set the oven to 250 degrees to preheat. Use a food processor to coarsely chop the almonds, being careful not to over-process and make a paste. Set these to the side.

Add the lemon zest and cinnamon to a medium bowl and mix. Add the beaten egg whites to this mixture and then stir in the lemon juice and honey. Beat until the ingredients are fully incorporated. Then, put the almond mixture in the bowl and blend well.

Take a piece of parchment paper and lay it on a baking sheet. Use a teaspoon to create mounds of the almond mixture. When you run out of dough, bake for 30 minutes. For easy removal, use a spatula to take the macaroons off the paper while they are slightly warm.

Chia Seed Pudding with Coconut and Pecans

This sweet recipe is easy to throw together and even so filling that you could eat it for breakfast. You can eat it about 2 hours after preparing but you should refrigerate overnight if you want the chia seeds especially soft.

Ingredients (for 4 servings)

- 2/3 cup chia seeds

- 3 cups full-fat coconut milk

- 1/3 cup unsweetened coconut (shredded)

- 1/3 cup pecans (chopped)

- 1 teaspoon raw honey

- 1 teaspoon vanilla extract

Instructions

Add the chia seeds to an airtight container or a mason jar and mix with the coconut milk, honey, and vanilla. When stirred well, seal and place in the refrigerator for at least 2 hours. Just before serving, stir in the coconut and pecans. Top with a few extra pieces of each to garnish.

Conclusion

Thank you again for Purchasing this book!

I hope this book was able to help you to realize some of your health goals using the Paleolithic Diet. Whether you are looking to lose weight or just to improve your overall health, the recipes and guidelines provided in this book can help you.

The next step is to clean the junk food out of your house and replace it with some of the nutrient-rich, wholesome foods to make the Paleo Diet recipes in the book. You have the knowledge, now the rest is up to you!

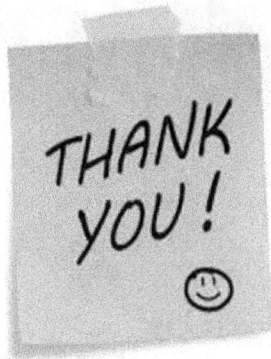